THE HANDBOOK OF PATIENT SAFETY COMPLIANCE

THE HANDBOOK OF PATIENT SAFETY COMPLIANCE

A Practical Guide for Health Care Organizations

Fay A. Rozovsky and James R. Woods Jr., Editors

Foreword by Maree Bellamy

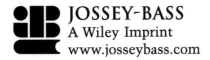

JOSSEY-BASS
A Wiley Imprint
www.josseybass.com

Published by Jossey-Bass
A Wiley Imprint
989 Market Street, San Francisco, CA 94103-1741   www.josseybass.com

Jossey-Bass books and products are available through most bookstores. To contact Jossey-Bass directly
call our Customer Care Department within the U.S. at 800-956-7739, outside the U.S. at 317-572-
399386 or fax 317-572-4002.

Jossey-Bass also publishes its books in a variety of electronic formats. Some content that appears in print
may not be available in electronic books.

Library of Congress Cataloging-in-Publication Data

The handbook of patient safety compliance : a practical guide for
  health care organizations / Fay A. Rozovsky and James R.
  Woods Jr., editors. — 1st ed.
    p. ; cm.
  Includes bibliographical references and index.
  ISBN 0-7879-6510-3 (alk. paper)
  1. Medical errors. I. Rozovsky, F. A. (Fay Adrienne), 1950-   .
II. Woods, James R., 1943-   .
  [DNLM: 1. Medical Errors—prevention & control. 2. Guideline
Adherence—organization & administration. 3. Medical Errors—legislation &
jurisprudence. 4. Safety Management—organization & administration.
  WB 100 H2363 2005]
R729.8.H36 2005
610—dc22   2004019606

Printed in the United States of America
FIRST EDITION
HB Printing   10 9 8 7 6 5 4 3 2 1

CONTENTS

FIGURES, TABLES, AND EXHIBITS

Figures

Tables

Exhibits

FOREWORD

Patient safety is making the transition from infancy and is entering a tumultuous adolescence, with all the resultant challenges.

Ensuring patient safety is the first critical step in improving quality of care. At all levels, health care workers make decisions every day involving patient safety. Patient safety is about protecting patients from incurring harm while they are receiving health care. It is an international issue. Although safe care has always been a priority, in recent times we have seen a growing realization of how unsafe care affects all the key stakeholder groups in the health care sector. Recognition and open acknowledgement have generated lively discussion as well as a search for solutions to the problem of unsafe care.

This book provides helpful perspectives on the evolution of patient safety, and suggestions for future activities geared to lessening the risk of harm. As discussed in this volume, several national studies, conducted in various countries, have identified unacceptable levels of adverse patient events, leading to the establishment of national and local strategies aimed at reducing the incidence of such events. Indeed, throughout the world new trends are emerging, including steps taken by organizations to appoint individuals with patient safety responsibilities, and the specific dedication of funds to patient safety projects and research. Many workshops and conferences have been held, and more are on the horizon. Standards for patient safety have been set by national groups and more are in the process of being set, and in some locations such standards are already an integral part of health care accreditation programs.

Accompanying this activity is a growing awareness of the importance of effective governance and risk management dedicated to the provision of safe health care services. In some settings the emphasis is on clinical risk management and clinical governance. In others it is on enterprise-wide or integrated risk management and health care governance strategies. As discussed throughout this book, national and international frameworks have been established. Examples also illustrate how risk management, patient safety, and quality improvement are intrinsically linked, rather than functioning as separate activities.

Many organizations find it difficult to strategize beyond the identification of error, risks, and adverse outcomes. It is essential that the right systems, protocols, standards, and incentives be in place to address the issues that are identified. This book provides a practical understanding of why patient safety is everyone's responsibility. It provides a framework for developing a patient safety program, effectively examining the adverse events that do occur, and ensuring that appropriate corrective and preventive actions are reviewed for effectiveness.

When patient safety is managed properly, it requires rigorous, forward thinking and encourages an organization to manage proactively rather than reactively. It requires a thorough understanding and appreciation of clinical and other processes in the health care organization, including knowledge of key business operations and the various standards and legislative requirements that have to be met. Patient safety must be managed continuously. The material provided in this book offers insight into a variety of patient safety tools and techniques and guidance for implementing these tools and techniques to manage patient safety in a consistent and systematic way. The underlying principles are generic, but each organization's unique environment determines which of these tools and techniques are likely to yield the greatest results in the local setting.

Although health care is a high-risk and complex industry, until recently it was lagging behind other industries that experience similar consumer safety expectations. We still have much more to learn from those groups about how to create an effective culture of safety, but the quest has begun. We now also have good information available from our own sector. The contributors to this book present resources and examples from health care as well as other industries to assist health care organizations to develop and implement patient safety programs successfully. Some of the most eminent patient safety specialists in the world are contributors to this volume. They have provided enormous depth and diversity of expertise to the wider health care community and to the development of innovative patient safety concepts.

This book also recognizes the impact of legislative and regulatory initiatives that have helped to shape contemporary patient safety efforts in the United States.

Equally apparent in some of the chapters is the need for legislative change, especially with regard to the use of patient safety and quality data in litigation involving health care professionals.

Going forward, the goal is to create a culture of safety across the continuum of care, supported by continuous improvement initiatives and effective governance and risk management strategies. Known already are many of the important ingredients in the recipe for patient safety. We know that the right culture can develop only where there is strong leadership from senior managers and boards of governance. These components must be accompanied by effective clinician involvement, using techniques that capture the enthusiasm of those who deliver care. And each of these elements must unite within the boundaries set by local medicolegal and regulatory conditions. A cohesive national strategy is imperative if we are to succeed in increasing patient safety. This book draws together important information and case studies that exemplify such initiatives, in the hope of stimulating practical interventions to further patient safety.

January 2005

Maree Bellamy
Australia

Note

Epigraph: J. DeRosier, E. Stalhandske, J. P. Bagian, and T. Nudell, "Using Healthcare Failure Modes and Effects Analysis: The VA National Center for Patient Safety's Prospective Risk Analysis System," *Joint Commission Journal on Quality Improvement,* 2002, 27(5), 248–267.

THE EDITORS

Fay A. Rozovsky has over twenty-five years of experience as a health care risk management consultant and attorney. She has lectured extensively and authored or coauthored over five hundred articles and several books including *Consent to Treatment: A Practical Guide; Clinical Trials and Human Research* (with Rodney Adams); and *What Do I Say? Communicating Intended or Unanticipated Outcomes in Obstetrics* (with James R. Woods Jr.). Her expertise in consent law has been recognized by several courts, including the U.S. Supreme Court in the *Cruzan* decision and the highest courts in Hawaii, Kentucky, West Virginia, and several other states. A graduate of Providence College, she received a JD degree from Boston College Law School and an MPH degree from the Harvard School of Public Health. She is an adjunct associate professor of Medical Humanities at the University of Rochester School of Medicine and Dentistry and an affiliate associate professor in the Department of Legal Medicine at the Medical College of Virginia. She is admitted to the practice of law in Florida and Massachusetts. A Distinguished Fellow of the American Society for Healthcare Risk Management, she is also a past president of the society. In 1998, she was awarded ASHRM's Distinguished Service Award, the highest honor bestowed on a member of ASHRM. Currently, she is the chair of the Professional Technical Advisory Committee for Hospitals of the Joint Commission on Accreditation of Healthcare Organizations.

James R. Woods Jr. is the Henry A. Thiede Professor and chair of the Department of Obstetrics and Gynecology at the University of Rochester School of Medicine, Rochester, New York. He completed medical school at the Bowman Gray School of Medicine, his residency in obstetrics and gynecology at Tripler Army Medical Center in Hawaii, and his perinatal fellowship at the UCLA School of Medicine. He has authored or coauthored over one hundred and forty articles on maternal-fetal medicine, maternal drug addiction, complications of pregnancy, and clinical research. His books include *What Do I Say? Communicating Intended or Unanticipated Events in Obstetrics* (with Fay A. Rozovsky). He has served as a regular member of an NIH Study Section (NIDA) and as guest editor for *Clinical Obstetrics and Gynecology* and *Obstetrics and Gynecology Clinics of North America.* In 1996, an endowed chair honoring Dr. Woods was established at the University of Rochester. He has been named in *Best Doctors in America* for many years, most recently 2003. He has lectured extensively on loss and grief in the medical setting. He has pioneered strategies for transforming some of the most challenging clinical interactions with patients after adverse outcomes into extraordinary opportunities for compassionate connection between clinicians and their patients and family members.

THE CONTRIBUTORS

Rodney K. Adams is an attorney with LeClair Ryan, A Professional Corporation, where he specializes in patient care issues and health care litigation. He represented several large hospitals and medical colleges in Chicago before moving to Richmond in 1991. He currently counsels and defends hospitals, nursing homes, physicians, and other health care providers in court and administrative forums, having defended more than thirty trials in Virginia. He has taught health law at the IIT-Kent College of Law and trial advocacy at the University of Richmond School of Law. He graduated from Millikin University; the University of Glasgow, Scotland (with an LLM degree in forensic medicine); and the University of Illinois College of Law. He is admitted to the state and federal courts of Virginia, District of Columbia, and Illinois. A member of the American Health Lawyers Association and the Virginia Association of Defense Attorneys, he serves on a hospital system bioethics committee and the board of directors for the St. Francis Home, a nonprofit assisted-living residence. He is cochair of the Medical Ethics Subcommittee, American Bar Association. A frequent speaker at state and national health care meetings, he is also the author of *Virginia Medical Law* (2000) and coauthor of *Clinical Trials and Human Research: A Practical Guide to Regulatory Compliance* (with Fay A. Rozovsky, 2003).

David M. Benjamin is a PhD-trained clinical pharmacologist and toxicologist and a nationally recognized scholar in legal medicine and the reduction of medication errors. He is adjunct assistant professor in the Department of Pharmacology and Experimental Therapeutics at Tufts University School of Medicine and is a guest lecturer at Harvard Medical School, Stetson University College of Law, and George Washington University Law School. A Fellow of the American College of Clinical Pharmacology, the American College of Legal Medicine, the American Academy of Forensic Sciences (Toxicology), and the American Society for Healthcare Risk Management, he has published or presented over 180 papers and has been featured on "Forensics Files" and Court-TV. He also serves on the editorial boards of the *Journal of Clinical Pharmacology* and the *Journal of Healthcare Risk Management.*

Christina W. Giles is the principal in Medical Staff Solutions, a consulting firm specializing in education and training medical staff administrative functions such as credentialing and privileging, assessment and development of medical staff governance documents, and survey preparation. She serves as an adviser to multiple medical staff publications, including Brownstone's *Credentialing and Peer Review Legal Insider;* and is a contributing editor to *The Handbook of Medical and Professional Staff Management.* She is an instructor for El Centro College's Medical Staff Services associate's degree program and has presented nationally on such topics as accreditation preparation, credentialing, privileging, and medical staff office management. She is a certified professional medical services management (CPMSM) and holds an MS degree.

Mark A. Kadzielski is the partner in charge of the West Coast Health Law Practice at Fulbright & Jaworski LLP. His practice focuses on the representation of hospitals, medical staffs, managed care enterprises, and institutional and individual health care providers throughout the United States in a broad spectrum of matters, including governmental regulatory investigations, managed care, credentialing, licensing, medical staff bylaws, Joint Commission accreditation and Medicare certification. He speaks and publishes frequently on matters of health law. He has been selected through peer evaluations for inclusion in the healthcare law section of *The Best Lawyers in America* for the past several years. He has served on the board of directors of both the American Academy of Healthcare Attorneys and the American Health Lawyers Association. He has also served on many advisory bodies in the healthcare industry. He earned his JD degree from the University of Pennsylvania Law School.

Susan Durbin Kinter is director of claims, litigation and risk management with the Maryland Medicine Comprehensive Insurance Program, a joint venture between the University of Maryland Medical System and University Physicians, Inc. Prior to joining the Maryland Medicine Comprehensive Insurance Program, she was an associate with Miles & Stockbridge, P.C., where her practice focused on medical malpractice defense litigation. She holds an RN degree, and she received her JD degree from the University of Maryland School of Law and her BSN degree from Michigan State University. She is a member of the American Society for Healthcare Risk Management, the Maryland Society for Healthcare Risk Management, and the Maryland Bar Association.

Robert J. Latino is executive vice president of strategic development for Reliability Center, Inc. (RCI). RCI is a consulting firm specializing in improving equipment, process, and human reliability. He has been facilitating RCA, FMEA, and OA analyses with his Fortune 500 clientele around the world for twenty years and has taught over 10,000 students in the PROACT Methodology, resulting in billions of dollars in documented savings. He has spent the last four years doing research on the health care culture as it contrasts to the industrial culture, in order to make appropriate modifications to methodologies and successfully bridge the proactive technologies from industry to health care. He is a coauthor of *Root Cause Analysis: Improving Performance for Bottom Line Results* (with Kenneth Latino, 2002) and a contributor to *Error Reduction in Healthcare: A Systems Approach to Improving Patient Safety* (1999). He has been published in numerous trade magazines and journals on the topics of RCA, FMEA, and OA and is also a frequent speaker on these topics at trade meetings and conferences. He received his bachelor's degree in business administration and management from Virginia Commonwealth University.

Jane C. McConnell is executive director of the Maryland Medicine Comprehensive Insurance Program, a joint venture between the University of Maryland Medical System and University Physicians, Inc. Her past positions include vice president, insurance and risk management, for the Franciscan Sisters of Allegheny Health System, Inc. in Tampa, Florida, vice president for risk management for FOJP Service Corporation in New York City, deputy director of the New York County Professional Review Organization, director of nursing at the Brooklyn Cumberland Medical Center, and director of quality assurance with the New York City Health Department. She received her JD degree from Fordham University School of Law, two master's degrees including an MBA degree from New York University, an RN degree from St. Vincent's Hospital in New York, and an Associate in Risk Management designation from the Insurance Institute of America. She is a past president of the American Society for Healthcare Risk Management and a member of the Maryland Society for Healthcare Risk Management and the American Bar Association.

Lara E. Parkin is an associate with the Health Care Practice group in Fulbright & Jaworski's Washington, D.C., office. Her practice focuses on litigation defense of pharmaceutical companies and regulatory matters involving the protection of human subjects in research. She received her BS degree with highest honors from the Florida Institute of Technology and her JD degree with high honors from the University of Florida, where she was managing editor of the *Journal of Law and Public Policy*. She is a member of the Virginia and District of Columbia bars.

Pamela L. Popp has over twenty years of health care risk and claims management experience. She will serve as president in 2005 for the American Society for Healthcare Risk Management (ASHRM). She is also on the board of directors, and serving as president, for the AHA Certification Center, which develops and administers the Certified Professional in Healthcare Risk Management (CPHRM) exam. She has held leadership positions in local, state, and national risk management organizations throughout her career. She obtained her bachelor's degree from Truman University, her M.A. degree from Webster University, and her JD degree from St. Louis University School of Law, and she is a Certified Professional in Healthcare Risk Management and a Fellow of ASHRM.

Peter J. Pronovost is a practicing anesthesiologist and critical care physician, a lecturer, a patient safety researcher, and leader. He is associate professor in the Departments of Anesthesiology and Critical Care Medicine and Surgery in the School of Medicine, Nursing in the School of Nursing and Health Policy and Management in the Bloomberg School of Public Health at the Johns Hopkins University. He has written more than 100 articles and chapters in the fields of patient safety, intensive care unit (ICU) care, quality health care, and evidence-based medicine. Within the Johns Hopkins community he is medical director for the Center for Innovations in Quality Patient Care and cochairs the hospital's Patient Safety Committee. Nationwide, he is chair of the ICU Advisory Panel for Quality Measures for the Joint Commission on Accreditation of Healthcare Organizations and chair of the ICU Physician Staffing Committee for the Leapfrog Group, is helping lead an effort to develop the ideal ICU design with the Institute for Healthcare Improvement, and is developing standards for ICU quality nationwide. He is currently leading two large, nationwide safety projects, funded by the Agency for Healthcare Research and Quality. In the first he is implementing an error-reporting system in 30 ICUs in the United States. In the second he is working with the Keystone Center for Patient Safety and Quality at the MHA Health Foundation to improve care in over 107 ICUs in the state of Michigan. His evaluation of the association between ICU organizational characteristics and outcomes formed the basis for the Leapfrog Group's ICU purchasing specification. In addition to his MD degree, he holds a PhD degree in clinical investigation from the Johns Hopkins Graduate Training Program in Clinical Investigation at the Bloomberg School of Public Health.

Frederick Robinson is the partner in charge of the Health Law Practice in Fulbright & Jaworski's Washington, D.C., office. His cases cover all phases of trial and appellate practice in both criminal and civil cases, including *qui tam*, or "whistle-blower," lawsuits under the federal False Claims Act, and represents major corporations and their officers in white-collar criminal cases. He also assists health care providers with the creation and implementation of corporate compliance programs and with voluntary disclosure matters. He has written numerous articles and is a regular speaker at seminars and conferences regarding health care compliance matters. He graduated with honors from Duke University School of Law in 1982 and is admitted to the Maryland and District of Columbia bars.

John P. Santell is director of educational program initiatives at the United States Pharmacopeia (USP) Center for the Advancement of Patient Safety, developing programs and publications to advance the scientific understanding of medication errors. He uses data collected through USP's two medication error-reporting programs—MEDMARX and the Medication Errors Reporting (MER) programs—to develop regular informative articles for several journals for health professionals. He is also the editor of *CAPSLink*, an e-newsletter that delivers the latest information and research on patient safety issues. Prior to taking his current position, he spent nine years with the American Society of Health-System Pharmacists (ASHP) as director, Center on Pharmacy Practice Management. His practice work experience also includes eleven years of hospital pharmacy positions, including director of pharmacy. He has extensively researched, authored, and published articles and made numerous presentations on topics related to patient safety and is a member of the ASHP and the Federation of International Pharmacy. A registered pharmacist, he earned his B.S. degree in pharmacy from Duquesne University and his M.S. degree from Ohio State University, and completed a two-year, ASHP-accredited residency in hospital pharmacy administration, also at Ohio State.

Ronni P. Solomon is executive vice president and general counsel of ECRI, a health services research agency in suburban Philadelphia that focuses on patient safety, evidence-based medicine, and health care technology. She has over twenty years of experience in developing and leading initiatives for both the public and private sectors on patient safety, adverse-event reporting systems, clinical guidelines development, quality assessments, and risk management in the United states and internationally. She has lectured extensively and authored numerous book chapters and articles on these topics. She received her JD degree from Widener University School of Law and completed undergraduate studies at Temple University.

THE HANDBOOK OF PATIENT
SAFETY COMPLIANCE

CHAPTER ONE

PATIENT SAFETY

Crossing the Chasm from Legal and Regulatory Compliance

Fay A. Rozovsky

The concept of *patient safety* caught mainstream attention with the publication of *To Err Is Human: Building a Safer Health System* (Kohn, Corrigan, and Donaldson, 2000). This Institute of Medicine (IOM) report captured worldwide attention with the suggestion that every year, 44,000 to 98,000 Americans lose their lives to medical error, a startling statistic. The data suggested that health care took more lives than those lost to motor vehicle accidents, breast cancer, AIDS, and workplace accidents. The report suggested that these deaths were due largely to bad systems in American health care. Regulatory and market-based strategies were offered in the IOM report, along with a goal of at least a 50 percent reduction in medical errors over a five-year period.

Two major themes emerged in *To Err Is Human:* that medical error is a systemic problem and that concerns about liability make health care systems hesitant to report errors. Yet without such information the health care field cannot learn effectively about mistakes and make positive changes.

Federal agencies responded with a report that delineated a number of recommendations for implementing the strategies discussed in *To Err Is Human.* The Quality Interagency Coordination Task Force report (QuIC, 2000) outlined a number of measures intended to effect positive change. At the state level, a number of jurisdictions have enacted legislation with the goal of improving patient safety. This legislation has taken many forms, from laws about voluntary and mandatory reporting of medical errors and adverse events (for example, in

Florida, New York, and Pennsylvania[1]) (Flowers and Riley, 2001) to laws designed to encourage disclosure (for example, in Colorado[2]) to laws that set nurse-patient ratios (for example, in California[3]).

Systemic change has also been provoked by private organizations, associations, and accreditation bodies. Medical residency programs must now comply with well-defined parameters for the number of hours of work that program participants may perform.[4] Patient safety indicators called *never events* have been promoted by the National Quality Forum (NQF).[5] Additionally, the Joint Commission on Accreditation of Healthcare Organizations (JCAHO) has put in place a host of standards designed to enhance patient safety along the continuum of care (see, for example, JCAHO, 2004).

Notwithstanding this mosaic of federal and state laws and private initiatives, patient safety seems an elusive goal. That this is the case is reflected in subsequent reports from the IOM, data from other groups that collect information on medication errors, and case law reports. Frustration with persistent patient safety concerns has resulted in some rethinking about what can be done to reduce medical error. Moving from an approach premised on *systemic* change to more individual-based accountability is one step in this regard. Redesigning laws that address evidentiary protection is another area of serious consideration.

Clearly, *patient safety* is an evolving concept in contemporary health care. The terms that define patient safety continue to undergo change. Care providers, lawyers, and public policy professionals grapple with what can be done to bridge the chasm between the goal of patient safety on the one hand and on the other the legal and regulatory environment that must be put in place to promote significant reduction in medical error.

Terms That Define Patient Safety

In its recent report titled *Patient Safety: Achieving a New Standard for Care*, the Institute of Medicine pointed out that the patient safety field needs a standardized terminology to facilitate data aggregation (IOM, 2004). Absent a common taxonomy with terms that all can use, and absent a standardized format for obtaining and reporting data, the field will be hard pressed to learn and to improve systems. The lack of a coherent taxonomy means that health care organizations spend too much effort comparing apples to oranges rather than apples to apples and oranges to oranges. The lack of standardized information sets is ironic in a field driven by data. The reality is that an error barely averted might be a *near miss* at one health care organization and a *good catch* at another facility.

In *Patient Safety*, the IOM calls for a streamlined approach. If this approach is accepted, the health care field would use the HL7 Clinical Document Architecture format, which enables a user to incorporate a narrative section within the framework of a standardized taxonomy of terms. As new terminology is identified, it would be incorporated using the Systemized Nomenclature of Human and Veterinary Medicine or SNOMED CT. To facilitate use of this common ground of patient safety terminology, the National Library of Medicine would be funded to maintain and distribute the taxonomy. The World Health Organization would be encouraged to enhance the International Classification of Diseases (ICD) 9/10-CM E-codes to permit collection of information on adverse events. This would enable international comparisons in the patient safety arena.

From a legal and regulatory standpoint the 2004 IOM report portends new legal concerns. It includes suggestions about delineating omissions and commissions in medical error. It suggests employing both *primary* and *secondary* event types. The latter could be significant in litigation. Depending on the infrastructure of the taxonomy and the way in which these terms are used in a legal setting, these primary and secondary event types might translate into contributory negligence or comparative negligence if part of the accountability for an adverse event is ascribed to the patient or family caregiver. At a more fundamental legal level the taxonomy might also be used out of context by lawyers representing aggrieved patients. Terms like *near miss, risk assessment index,* and *omission* and *commission* could be portrayed in an electronic display before a jury and make more difficult for the defense the task of presenting factual information about what transpired in the occurrence.

There is a need for a consistent taxonomy of terms in the patient safety arena. There is a concomitant need for standardized data sets and other information with which to develop practical methods for error reduction. Using SNOMED CT and refreshing the content of ICD-9/10-CM E-codes are good starts. However, the developmental phase of the process needs to be schooled by an understanding of the ways the taxonomy and data may be used for other purposes. Medical malpractice litigation is but one example. The taxonomy and data might also be used in terminations of agreements between health care facilities and health plans, professional licensure proceedings, and regulatory inquiries by federal funding sources. If the terminology can be easily taken out of context and used for other purposes, the recoil may be a reluctance to use it. These concerns can be avoided. In developing the taxonomy and the data sets, several steps can be taken to ensure proper use:

- The passage of legislation and regulations defining specific and limited uses of the taxonomy for purposes of patient safety and medical error reduction
- The involvement of risk management professionals and health care attorneys in the process of developing a coherent, neutral taxonomy of terms

- The inclusion of data weighting and stratification to ensure accurate use of the information and apple-to-apple comparisons
- Restrictions on using data gathered in the reporting process as evidence in certain circumstances, including litigation
- The education of the public and the media on how to interpret the results of data gleaned from the process

Whether or not these strategies are implemented, health care organizations can take positive steps to limit potential harm from embracing a standardized taxonomy of terms and data aggregation for patient safety. Working with legal counsel, risk management, and health information professionals, senior leadership can implement safeguards with respect to

- Collecting data
- Applying terminology
- Using and explaining information in reports
- Educating staff
- Educating media
- Explaining information to the community

By taking such steps, health care facilities can preempt out-of-context reports or other information use. Staff will know what the data and reports mean within the framework of the health care organization. Legal counsel defending the organization will have a solid foundation from which to respond to out-of-context use of the data by plaintiffs' counsel or those representing the government in an adjudicatory proceeding. The following example demonstrates this approach:

A hospital CEO learns that a patient safety report has received notoriety in the local press. The headline reads, "Falls out of control at local hospital." The article describes the findings of a patient safety project focused on medical-surgical falls. It highlights the fact that some 10 patients suffered injuries in postsurgical falls. What the article does not include are some very important data: the 10 falls occurred among a patient population of 5,500 identified as "at risk" for postsurgical falls. All the injuries involved bruises and contusions. There were no fractured limbs or internal injuries. Rather than a project that portrayed a disaster in patient care, the study was the culmination of a patient safety program for those at risk of falling in the twenty-four hours following inpatient surgery. The study had been conducted after the environment of care had been revamped and staff educated on fall avoidance. The number of falls had been reduced from 105 for a similar cohort a year earlier, when 3 patients had suffered pelvic and wrist fractures and 2 had sustained concussions. Instead of a hospital "out of control" on falls, the study revealed a major victory in patient safety.

Although the CEO has the public relations officer do some damage control, the public is irate. When confronted with the truth, the newspaper apologizes and promises to help unwind the false impression it created in its headline and story. The newspaper editor says that a reporter saw a storyboard on the study on a hospital bulletin board and misunderstood the information.

The lesson learned was this: when dealing with a new initiative (such as a patient safety taxonomy and data aggregation tool), make certain that all consumers of the information understand what they are reading and how to use the information.

The Legal and Regulatory Influences Constraining Patient Safety: Evidentiary Protection

A number of initiatives are underway to encourage the sharing of adverse-event information among health care organizations. The goal is to learn from these situations in order to reduce the likelihood of repetitions that could result in catastrophic injury. Few would dispute the importance of this laudable goal. Avoiding needless patient injuries while improving quality outcomes of care is a common theme found in acute care and other health care facilities. Aside from technical issues such as the taxonomy of terms and standardized data sets, some legal and regulatory constraints exist:

- Legal requirements for confidentiality of data
- Concern that identifying an adverse event will be tantamount to an admission of liability
- Fear that sharing data outside the facility will be seen as a voluntary relinquishment of evidentiary protection under applicable state laws
- Fear that providing data will mean a physician is blamed for the event and will result in corrective action under medical staff bylaws
- Fear that providing data will mean that a nurse or pharmacist is disciplined or fired under the facility's employment requirements

Some may question whether these are substantive legal concerns or merely speculation engendered by a lack of understanding of the law. Addressing each item individually puts these concerns in context.

Legal Requirements for Confidentiality of Data

As is discussed later in this book (Chapter Eleven), there is no uniform legal approach to maintaining confidentiality of adverse-event information. Although some states provide strong legal protections, others do not do so. Further, the application of state-based confidentiality laws varies within each jurisdiction for hospitals, for long-term care facilities, and for other types of health care organizations.

The absence of confidentiality protection at the federal level also reinforces a concern that adverse-event information could be used for purposes that do not promote patient safety. Indeed, even when adverse-event information is generated under the protection of a state law provision, if those data are then properly obtained by a federal agency as part of a focused review involving patient safety, the information will no longer be cloaked by the state-based confidentiality requirements. This potential reinforces concerns about sharing adverse-event information.

Concern That Identifying an Adverse Event Will Be Tantamount to an Admission of Liability

There are some observers who believe that the mere characterization of an outcome as an adverse event will be interpreted as an admission of culpability for a negligent act. The prospect of this risk serves as a deterrent to reporting of adverse events. Although this risk appears to be remote, it can be addressed with a practical strategy. Statements can be included in the policy and procedure that specify the intent of the adverse-event reporting process. The description of the intent should make it clear that identification of adverse events does not constitute an admission of culpability or constitute a negligent act. And a definition should be included that gives precision to the meaning of *adverse event*. Even if adverse-event data is considered discoverable and admissible as evidence of negligent care, the defense can use the policy and procedure to correct any misunderstandings about the nature and purpose of the information. Implementing this type of strategy can help address the concern that adverse-event data may be seen as evidence of negligence.

Fear That Sharing Data Outside the Facility Will Be Seen as a Voluntary Relinquishment of Evidentiary Protection Under Applicable State Laws

A legitimate concern is that adverse-event data sharing among various health care facilities might abrogate evidentiary protection. This concern is genuine in some states, and the response in those states may be to refrain from sharing adverse-event data.

However, another approach is to explore how certain data elements can be shared with other entities without fear of this type of evidentiary outcome. One strategy may be to include participants from other health care facilities as members of the peer review or quality improvement process under which the data are generated and evaluated. The review of the data is enriched by including others as members of the protected review process, yet the data remain within the organization rather than migrating. Additional steps are needed to make this a practical option. Legal counsel need to examine carefully the specifics of state law to make certain that this approach will work. Additionally, bylaws, policies, and procedures of the facility may need to be amended to provide for others to participate in the review process. The review will have to be done at the data-generating organization.

Ideally, enhanced peer review and quality improvement laws will remove the need for employing such an option. Nonetheless, for those who want to share adverse-event information to improve patient safety, this may be a practical step.

Fear That Providing Data Will Mean a Physician Is Blamed for the Event and Will Result in Corrective Action Under Medical Staff Bylaws

Many physicians are concerned that adverse-event data may be used to affix blame on them, a concern that is incongruent with the underlying *systems* philosophy of the patient safety movement. Those who share this concern fear that a blaming mentality will have serious repercussions, including corrective action within the health care organization and possible licensure proceedings through the auspices of the state board regulating the practice of medicine.

There is a difference between a punitive approach and an accountability philosophy in patient safety. Assigning responsibility to physicians or blaming physicians for adverse outcomes does not recognize that most untoward events are the culmination of several systemic failures that coalesce in failure. It is easier to point a finger at some physicians than it is to tease out which system components failed and how these problems can be corrected.

Since the late 1990s, efforts have been underway to move from the blaming mentality. This initiative has required health care organizations to change their intrinsic culture and their approach to error prevention and reduction. However, as the notion of blamelessness gained notoriety, it was realized that there still needs to be room for individual responsibility. Although system components may fail and result in patients' receiving the wrong medication, the fact remains that some health care professionals have individual accountability for these adverse outcomes. That hospitals enable clinically incompetent doctors to continue to prescribe wrong medications does not detract from the fact that such care providers bear individual responsibility for their actions. With the evolution of the patient safety movement, two important factors have emerged regarding data and accountability. One is that data are imperative for our understanding of why systems fail and how improvements can be made to promote safety. The other is that these data can be used not to punish but to foster individual accountability for patient safety.

Data also can lead to the suspension or revocation of physicians' privileges. When this happens, health care organizations reinforce the fear that adverse-event data will be used to punish doctors. In more enlightened health care organizations, adverse-event data drive efforts to help physicians understand where they have deficiencies and to help them achieve quality, safe patient care. This may be accomplished through intense in-service education, clinical coursework at other facilities, or one-to-one mentoring. Achieving and maintaining compliance with established safety parameters introduces an accountability approach. It does not involve the use of a big stick to punish for bad outcomes.

Health care organizations are obliged to report certain types of corrective action to state licensure agencies. Independently, dissatisfied patients may file complaints with these agencies. They may seek sanctions or licensure revocation for some physicians. Adverse-event data could be used to make the case for taking such actions. Given the framework in which licensing bodies must operate, they have limited recourse to avoid such responses. The prospect of such regulatory action reinforces the concern of some physicians about the uses of adverse-outcome data. In reality few types of events trigger reports to licensure agencies. Significant evidence must be presented by aggrieved patients to generate responses from licensure agencies. It also takes a substantial amount of information on serious outcomes to compel the use of corrective actions in health care organizations. Thus, on balance, there is a low risk that collecting and using adverse-event data will result in corrective action or licensure activity against physicians.

Fear That Providing Data Will Mean a Nurse or Pharmacist Is Disciplined or Fired Under the Facility's Employment Requirements

The nursing profession sometimes is labeled as one that will "eat its own" for errors or omissions that result in patient injury. Nurses have been seen as having less tolerance for clinical mistakes than physicians do. In the patient safety arena, nurses and pharmacists share the light of scrutiny with physicians. As the culture of blamelessness emerged, some thought it would work to dispel the idea of severe retribution against nurses for serious errors. The case of Betsy Lehman was emblematic of this approach. In the aftermath of a catastrophic medication error at Dana Farber Cancer Institute, detailed evaluations were conducted by JCAHO and the Massachusetts Department of Health. The facility took responsibility for a series of system failures that culminated in the death of a patient from an overdose of medication. The facility made clear that it did not hold the nurses who cared for the patient accountable for the medication error.

A few years later, however, the fear of retribution for adverse outcomes reemerged when the Board of Registration in Nursing decided to pursue sanctions against eighteen nurses involved in this 1994 event that led to the death of Betsy Lehman. The Massachusetts Nurses Association and the Massachusetts Organization of Nurse Executives took a public stand in the hope of persuading the board not to take action against these nurses: "While we believe nurses should and must be held accountable for the safety of their patients and for the integrity of their practice, no nurse should suffer consequences for systemic failures beyond their control" (Massachusetts Nurses Association, 1999). The point made by the Massachusetts Nurses Association is as compelling for pharmacists and other regulated health care professionals. Accountability and integrity are at the core of patient safety. Systemic failures that they cannot control should not trigger disciplinary action. By creating an institutional culture premised on accountability and individual responsibility, health care organizations can put a framework in place that nurtures adverse-event reporting.

Regulatory bodies must respond to their legislative mandates. Public policy changes and legislative reform will be necessary. In the interim the use of internal review mechanisms and external evaluations—like those in the Betsy Lehman case—actually may enhance the framework for adverse-event reporting. That institutions demonstrate that they are accountable and that their employees are held to a similar standard may limit professional disciplinary action by licensing boards to those instances in which such activity is warranted.

Perhaps the most important step for deflecting all the concerns discussed here is the enactment of legislation that fosters data gathering and sharing of adverse-event information. If this legislation is written in a way that creates incentives for reporting and using such information, health care organizations and professionals can glean ideas for reducing and preventing errors. Until that time, practical steps can be taken to address the legitimate concerns of care providers who fear retribution.

The Legal Concepts of Standards of Care and Patient Safety

The law is driven by the concept of standards. Legislation and regulations set minimum requirements for care providers to follow. This does not preclude providers from setting higher standards of performance. Those higher standards might arise from a variety of sources, including learned journals or treatises, position statements from a specialty medical college or nursing organization, or internal policies and procedures developed by health care organizations. Sometimes health care entities transform clinical guidelines developed as a pathway for patient care into a standard of care. The health care field shares this legal construct with many other professional groups. Plumbers, electricians, and professional engineers, for example, also are expected to conduct themselves in accordance with recognized standards of care. Some of these standards emanate from legislation or regulations. Others are generated by national trade associations.

Standards play a key role in the law. A failure to meet established standards may be the basis for terminating a contract. A failure to meet standards may trigger the withholding of payment for services in industry or in the health care field. It also may be the basis for professional liability claims and, in particular, medical malpractice litigation. Understanding the significance of standards puts into context some of the forces influencing the patient safety movement.

The Legal Concept of Standards

Standards are usually set at a minimal level of performance. Thus, if a nurse holds himself out as a *specialist* in cardiac rehabilitation nursing, he will be expected to live up to the standards of a person with those qualifications. His failure to do so can have serious consequences. His employment may be premised on his meeting the standards for such a nurse specialist. Performance that does not meet that level could result in termination of employment. If the nurse has held himself out to be a specialist and does not perform accordingly, with the result being foreseeable injury to a patient, the situation might lead to a professional liability action. As the bar on standards is raised, the level of expected performance is increased. If this nurse held himself out as a nonspecialist in nursing, there might then be no basis for such a claim. As long as the nurse met the standards for an average, reasonable, prudent nurse in the same or similar circumstance, a plaintiff would be hard pressed to demonstrate all the requisite elements of a claim for professional liability.

For many of the procedures in health care, there are now guidelines, pronouncements, and clinical pathways to drive the performance of individual care providers. For example, there is more than one correct approach to performing gastric bypass, and there are competing dietary regimens for weight reduction. The law has evolved to the point that it will not pick and choose among equally valid standards of care. If the evidence presented suggests that two or more differing methodologies are equally acceptable, it is not for a court to say that one is better than the others. That a patient has sustained a bad outcome as a result of a physician's following one standard of care and not another does not automatically suggest that the doctor was culpable of medical malpractice. As long as it can be shown that the standards of care were comparable, there can be no finding of negligence. Quite a different outcome can occur when a care provider follows a standard that is below the minimum level of expected performance. If, for example, a surgeon uses a technique long since rejected by the field and as a consequence the patient is harmed, there would be a strong basis for a claim.

However, as described earlier, when a care provider holds herself out as one who performs at a higher level, she will be measured by that standard. For example, a neurosurgeon might hold herself out as an expert in high-risk laminectomies. Relying on this fact, a patient agrees to have the neurosurgeon perform this surgery. The patient sustains a permanent disability as a consequence of the laminectomy, and it is shown that this injury was the result of the neurosurgeon performing in a substandard manner and not at the level of an expert in such high-risk procedures. The result is that the neurosurgeon will be held to the higher standard of care because she clearly presented herself as one who performed at that elevated level of surgical expertise.

Proving which standard is the applicable standard is a function of evidence. Information is drawn from experts. It is drawn from data found in peer-reviewed studies, journals, and books. It also is found in standards from contracts and applicable legislation and regulations.

Standards are applied in the context of a given circumstance. This is a key point in the law. The expected level of care or standard in an emergency department may not be applicable in the context of a train derailment in which dozens of injured passengers need immediate care in an open field. The applicability of the standard is adjusted to the circumstances.

Finally, the law anticipates that standards will change over time. In the context of negligence litigation, however, the standard of care is measured by what was expected at the time of the event. Although today the use of a tourniquet is rejected in first-responder aid for a snakebite, in years past it was the acceptable standard of care. A lawsuit brought in 2003 for alleged negligent use of a tourniquet in 1999 would involve the application of the clinical standards in existence at the time of the snakebite.

These points are of particularly significant in the arena of patient safety. As clinical pathways, guidelines, and statistical process controls (SPCs) emerge to drive clinical care, the connection with standards must be considered from a legal and regulatory perspective.

The Legal Significance of a Standard in Patient Safety

For the plaintiffs' bar, the often-quoted Gertrude Stein phrase "Rose is a rose is a rose is a rose" is particularly relevant with respect to patient safety standards. Legal counsel are adept at convincing juries that what is showcased as a "goal" or a "guideline" is a façade for a standard of care. The task of the defense is to disabuse juries from the idea that this is the case. Sometimes the defense is not successful in doing so.

Everyone shares the hope that the health care field will eliminate patient injuries and deaths from medical error. Public policy makers, leaders in the health care field, and care providers are striving for systems and processes that will reach this level of performance. However, in the drive to accomplish this lofty objective, many practical issues with profound legal ramifications must be considered.

When a state or a national trade association or accrediting body adopts a patient safety goal or standard, that goal or standard is expected to have broad application. The California law requiring certain minimum nurse-patient staffing ratios is a good illustration. Reducing the number of patients for whom a nurse is expected to provide care is seen as reducing the opportunity for errors and increasing safe outcomes. The nurse-patient ratio law has created a patient safety standard. The expectation has been set that health care facilities in California will meet this legal standard of care. The failure to do so can trigger a number of legal consequences. The reality is that health care facilities in California are facing the same nurse shortage as facilities across the rest of the country. Even if the California facilities could afford the staffing increase, finding the qualified personnel is a challenge.

The point is that the downstream consequences of establishing a standard should be considered carefully. The financial, material, and personnel requirements must be contemplated whether the standard is the result of legislation or regulation or of a pronouncement by a voluntary trade association. A more practical approach might be to adopt more than one standard or process for addressing each specific target in patient safety.

Providing latitude in terms of equipment, personnel, medication, and process would give health care organizations and professionals the leeway needed to meet such patient safety targets. The content of disparate standards can be evidence based. Thus what may work for a 350-bed, tertiary, acute care facility may not be the same as what works for a critical access hospital. Along with differing evidence-based criteria, accountability can be built in to measure performance. Outcomes that demonstrate achievement of recognized patient safety targets could become paramount, not a regimented process or standard that does not fit all care settings.

In January 2003, the federal government published a new standard that focused on provider efforts for patient safety. Part of the Conditions of Participation in Medicare and Medicaid for Hospitals, this quality assessment and performance improvement (QAPI) regulation reinforces the point that the notion of patient safety is not only about process. It is also about outcomes involving quality, safe care. As stated in the preamble to the QAPI regulation: "We are requiring that a hospital's QAPI program be an ongoing program that shows measurable improvement in indicators for which there is evidence that they will improve health outcomes and identify and reduce medical errors" (68 *Fed. Reg.* 16, 3435–3455, Jan. 24, 2003). The QAPI regulation is premised on accountability. It is also grounded on the reality that there must be some latitude for achieving and maintaining quality care. Absent is the idea that one size fits all. To this extent the regulation is consistent with the understanding that various approaches can be followed to achieve a common purpose: quality, safe care.

A Practical Approach to Dealing with Patient Safety Standards

Health care professionals and facilities face many challenges. Staffing shortages and low reimbursement rates confront those who must decide how to meet demands for technology enhancements and patient safety. Not meeting federal or state requirements is not an option, as that would be clear evidence of standards noncompliance. Within the framework of current resources, there are some practical measures for achieving and maintaining patient safety standards:

1. *Set priorities for patient safety standards.* Work on the key safety areas first.
2. *Set reasonable expectations.* Design standards, goals, and processes that can be achieved within the framework of existing personnel, equipment, and technology.
3. *Conduct failure modes and effects analysis on proposed standards.* Do a 360-degree analysis *before* launching a new standard or process. Take into account budget, equipment, staffing, insurance, and patient needs and complexity as well as other needs in the facility. Address bottlenecks or safety factors that arise from the proposed standard or process.
4. *Field-test the patient safety standard or process.* Pilot the new standard or process to make certain it works within the environment of care. Identify and resolve problem areas.
5. *Educate.* Make certain that all personnel understand how to use the new standard or process. Use competency-based testing for this purpose.
6. *Monitor.* Use a surveillance approach to determine whether the revised process is working as anticipated over time.
7. *Ongoing improvement.* Continuously monitor changes in the field, including evidence-based outcome data that might point to needed changes to the standard or process. Consider as well new staffing initiatives, the introduction of new equipment, and new regulations or medications that might necessitate changes to the standard or process.
8. *Follow a consistent approach.* Use one type of comprehensive analysis to evaluate a patient safety standard or process.
9. *Document the process.* Use a clear, understandable method for recording how the standard or process was developed, implemented, and improved.
10. *Be receptive to multiple standards or processes.* Accommodate different pathways or standards for achieving quality, safe patient care.

Finally, health care organizations need to develop and employ an understandable taxonomy of terms. Universally used definitions are as necessary for such words as *error, near miss,* and *adverse event* as they are for such words as *standard.* The glossary found in the 2004 IOM report is a good starting point. Involving legal counsel and the organization's risk management professional in the development of the taxonomy may help to avert potential liability concerns. Ultimately, a consistent methodology and uniform meanings for terms should help propel the development of patient safety standards and measures.

Notes

1. See *Florida Statutes* § 395.0197 (2001) as amended (which requires the timely reporting of events termed *Code 15*); the Medical Care Availability and Reduction of Error (MCARE) Act of 2002, Pennsylvania Public Law 154, No. 13, § 308 *et seq.* (which includes a patient disclosure provision); and New York Patient Occurrence Reporting and Tracking System (NYPORTS), N.Y. Public Health Law § 2805-1 (1998) as amended (which requires hospitals in New York to report certain types of events on an Internet-based system).
2. § 13-25-135 of the *Colorado Revised Statutes* (2003) makes it clear that in a civil proceeding involving an unanticipated outcome of medical care, any apology or expression of sympathy by a health care professional is inadmissible as evidence of admission of liability by the health care professional.
3. The California Business & Professions Act § 2725.3 (effective 2004) and the *California Health Safety Code* § 1276.4 (effective 2004) set minimum staff ratios for nurses in California hospitals.
4. The Residency Review Committee Program of the Accreditation Council for Graduate Medical Education, a private organization that accredits over 7,500 residency education programs, limits resident duty to eighty hours per week (see http://www.acgme.org).
5. The National Quality Forum's membership includes a number of well-known organizations, and NQF's list of twenty-seven serious reportable events has been used in legislation. For example, Minnesota has incorporated this list into its Adverse Health Care Events Reporting Law §§ 144.706–144.7069 (2003).

References

Flowers, L., and Riley, T. *State-Based Mandatory Reporting of Medical Errors: An Analysis of the Legal and Policy Issues.* Portland, Maine: National Academy for State Health Policy, 2001.

Institute of Medicine. *Patient Safety: Achieving a New Standard for Care.* Washington, D.C.: National Academies Press, 2004.

Joint Commission on Accreditation of Healthcare Organizations. *2004 Comprehensive Accreditation Manual for Hospitals: The Official Handbook.* Oakbrook Terrace, Ill.: Joint Commission on Accreditation of Healthcare Organizations, 2004.

Kohn, L. T., Corrigan, J. M., and Donaldson, M. S. (eds.). *To Err Is Human: Building a Safer Health System*. Washington, D.C.: National Academies Press, 2000.

Massachusetts Nurses Association. "MNA Statement Regarding Board of Registration in Nursing Sanctions of Dana Farber Nurses." [http://www.massnurses.org/News/1999/990400/boardreg.htm]. May–June, 1999.

Quality Interagency Coordination Task Force. *Doing What Counts for Patient Safety: Federal Actions to Reduce Medical Errors and Their Impact*. Publication No. OM 00-0004. Rockville, Md.: Agency for Healthcare Research and Quality, Feb. 2000.

CHAPTER TWO

PATIENT SAFETY LAWS
AND REGULATIONS

Ronni P. Solomon

Patient safety laws and regulations are not new. The number and intensity have increased dramatically, however, in the wake of the two seminal reports of the Institute of Medicine (IOM) on patient safety, *To Err Is Human* and *Crossing the Quality Chasm* (Kohn, Corrigan, and Donaldson, 2000; IOM, 2001). These reports present several recommendations for ways in which the legal system should support efforts to reduce preventable medical errors, enhance public account- ability, develop a knowledge base on medical errors, and facilitate culture change in health care organizations in order to promote the recognition of errors and improve patient safety. In the wake of these reports, many states adopted laws on patient safety, and new bills continue to proliferate in state legislatures as well as in Washington, D.C. The current crisis in medical malpractice insurance has spurred even more state action, some of which attempts to integrate aspects of tort reform with patient safety.

A third Institute of Medicine Report, issued in 2004, calls for all health care settings to establish comprehensive patient safety programs involving adverse- event and near-miss detection and analysis. New federal regulations on patient safety, issued by the Centers for Medicare & Medicaid Services (CMS), include *Conditions of Participation* that follow the recommendations of the IOM reports and call for quality assessment and performance improvement (see 42 *C.F.R.* § 482.21, 2003). The first version of the National Patient Safety Goals issued by the Joint Commission on Accreditation of Healthcare Organizations (JCAHO) became effective on January 1, 2003. These goals are revised and updated annually. Although they are not laws or regulations, they may ultimately be used in court as evidence of a standard of care in a medical malpractice case and thus may have important legal value.[1]

Unfortunately, many of the patient safety reforms spurred by the IOM reports are on a collision course with the current U.S. medical malpractice system (Studdert and Brennan, 2001). The patient safety movement encourages candor, disclosure, the learning of lessons, and systems improvement. The tort system encourages silence, adversity, and punishment. The patient safety movement searches for ways to focus on systems-related problems that contribute to the occurrence of errors and accidents in a complex environment. The tort system searches for ways to attribute errors and accidents to a single individual. Patient safety programs fix problems; the tort system fixes blame.

Traditional tort reform measures, such as abolition of the collateral source rule, caps on damages, mandatory periodic instead of lump sum payments, and shortened statutes of limitations may help to ease the medical liability insurance crisis. For example, tort reform measures adopted in California's Medical Injury Compensation Reform Act (MICRA) in 1975 are often cited as a successful intervention in a state-level crisis marked by high insurance premiums, high defense costs, carriers leaving the market, and physicians leaving medical practice. According to some sources, such tort reform efforts keep liability insurance available, keep premiums down, and keep physicians in practice, which in turn help to ensure patient access to care. But regardless of success with keeping insurance premiums down, there is little if any evidence to show that tort reform has had a positive impact on patient safety by reducing medical error or adverse events.

Mandatory Reporting Systems

The IOM has stressed the importance of creating a culture in hospitals and other health care organizations that promotes identifying errors, evaluating the causes, and implementing remedial actions (Kohn, Corrigan, and Donaldson, 2000). It recognizes that mandatory reporting systems are one mechanism for accomplishing this goal. One IOM recommendation calls for Congress to require health care providers to report serious injuries and deaths to state governments. This reporting requirement would apply first to hospitals and ultimately extend to other institutional and ambulatory care delivery settings. Another IOM recommendation is that a new federal agency be established to, among other things, receive and analyze reports from the states. The IOM envisions that reports involving serious harm would be available to the public.

Although reporting systems are a fundamental link in many patient safety initiatives, it is important to recognize both their strengths and their weaknesses. They are useful as early warning systems and as sources of information on problems. This raises awareness of harm or potential harm caused by the health care system. However, the data collected through a reporting system are not ends in themselves and, without further study, do not provide reliable information on what causes harm or which methods can be used to prevent future harm. Causes still need to be understood and risk-reduction strategies still need to be developed. Moreover, these efforts might require sophisticated investigation techniques and specialized knowledge. In addition, reporting systems are often mistakenly perceived as a reliable indicator of the rate of adverse events. In reality, underreporting is the norm.

Mandatory reporting systems for adverse events are not new. Indeed, many were implemented before the publication of the first IOM report, which identified a number of states with mandatory systems. In 2002, the National Academy for State Health Policy (2004) identified twenty-two states with mandatory reporting programs.[2] Several states, such as New Jersey and Pennsylvania, have now expanded their patient safety reporting requirements. Although reporting systems may underpin the effort to promote patient safety interventions, their effectiveness has been reduced because medical professionals fear that reports will stimulate lawsuits, disciplinary proceedings, and adverse publicity. Lack of trust in the system leads to noncompliance. That is at least part of the reason underreporting is the norm. A 2001 study found that six states received more than one hundred reports annually (Rosenthal, Booth, Flowers, and Riley, 2001). In addition, organized medicine opposes mandatory reporting initiatives, arguing that the lack of confidentiality and legal protection would, in effect, increase the volume of litigation (see, for example, Reardon, 2000). Confidentiality has been a key factor in the debate. There is no federal legislation that protects reported data, although in 2002, federal protection legislation was proposed. State laws vary— from strong protection to vague protection to no protection at all. Even where statutory protection for peer review data exists, there is no guarantee that this protection will apply in all cases to a mandatory reporting system. Plaintiffs' attorneys often challenge peer review and other statutes that provide protection, and the courts have issued varying opinions. In fact, as mentioned earlier, the IOM has recommended that reports involving serious harm should be available to the public. Hospitals and organized medicine are concerned that documents developed to comply with patient safety laws and regulations might be discoverable and admissible in medical malpractice lawsuits, government enforcement actions, and disciplinary proceedings—in effect, an open invitation to the blame culture attendant to the tort system. Again, the tort system is at odds with a culture of openness and candor espoused by the IOM report.

The IOM has recommended that Congress pass federal legislation providing peer review protection for the near-miss data collected in voluntary reporting databases but not for the serious injury data contained in mandatory reporting databases. This dichotomy has been questioned. One could argue that there is a greater likelihood of legal action in cases where the harm is greater, because attorneys would be more likely to accept and litigate the case. Because medical professionals have more reason to fear litigation after a serious injury than after a minor one, it would follow that stronger protections designed to encourage disclosure would be needed for the former rather than the latter (O'Connell and Bryan, 2000).

Data reported or maintained as part of a mandatory reporting system will likely be of keen interest to a plaintiff's attorney in that this information might be highly relevant to a medical malpractice case against an individual provider or an institution. (For an excellent overview of the clashes between the IOM's recommendations and the current tort system's practices, see O'Connell and Bryan, 2000.) These data may be valuable even if patients' identities are not reported or attending physicians' names are not cited. For example, these data may apply in cases against an institution that allege various forms of corporate negligence occurred or that the institution had notice of a hazard but failed to take remedial action.

In 2002, Pennsylvania passed the Medical Care Availability and Reduction of Error Act (MCare), a law addressing the medical malpractice insurance crisis and encompassing reforms aimed at the legal system, the insurance industry, and patient safety. MCare places a cap on punitive damages, establishes a collateral source rule, and makes provisions for periodic payment of future medical expenses. It lowers the amount of mandatory professional liability, limits insurer liability, and restricts the ability to cancel liability insurance policies. The quid pro quo for these reforms is a broad set of patient safety requirements (discussed later in this chapter). Physicians, other health care workers and medical facilities are now required to report serious events to the Pennsylvania Health Department as well as to the newly established Patient Safety Authority, which in turn must contract with an outside agency to analyze the reports and make recommendations to improve patient safety.[3] Patients affected by a serious event in a medical facility must receive written notice of the event. Physicians and licensed health care workers are required to inform their licensing boards of any complaints or disciplinary or legal actions against them, and the state medical board has the enforcement authority to conduct independent investigations. Unlike laws in other states, the Pennsylvania law also requires that medical facilities report near misses to the Patient Safety Authority and that the data be analyzed by an independent entity. This comports with the IOM (2004) recommendation that encourages near-miss reporting and analysis systems because near misses are often precursors of adverse events and thus are opportunities for learning and prevention.

Anatomy of a Patient Safety Law: Compliance Tips

The first step in complying with legal and regulatory requirements on patient safety is to obtain and learn the applicable rules. The rules may be complex, and when that is the case, authoritative interpretive guidance should be obtained. Rules also change, and they may do so from state to state and even among state agencies within a state. Federal rules may vary from state rules. Thus it is important to establish a system for ongoing monitoring of regulatory and policy developments at the federal, state, and local levels.

In planning for implementation, it is important to anticipate potential barriers to compliance. This is usually an ongoing rather than one-time effort. Support from top leadership is key. Effective training of medical professionals and of staff at all levels of the institution on the requirements of the applicable rules is key. Clear policies, procedures, and review mechanisms should be established to support the effort.

Patient safety is an area of high interest to several branches of government and other stakeholders. Legislatures, governmental agencies, and accreditation agencies are taking an increasing role in enforcement. The judiciary, through medical malpractice and other civil lawsuits, will rule on cases involving alleged violation of patient safety laws and standards. Federal and state mandates and accreditation standards expect institutions to establish patient safety programs. These mandates are enforced through scheduled or unannounced inspections. Violations may mean substantial fines or may affect the institution's licensure or ability to participate in federally funded programs.

Many states have a mandatory reporting system, and the requirements vary in terms of the types of events that must be reported, the protections afforded, and the follow-up actions taken by state regulators. The example I will focus on here, introduced earlier in this chapter, is Pennsylvania's Medical Care Availability and Reduction of Error Act, which was signed into law on March 20, 2002. MCare attempts to address several facets of the state's medical liability crisis, such as tort reform, insurance reform, and patient safety. The patient safety provisions are intended to reduce and eliminate medical errors by identifying problems and implementing solutions that promote patient safety.

Who is covered? MCare requirements apply to certain types of health care providers and organizations: ambulatory surgical facilities, birthing centers, behavioral health facilities, and hospitals.

What are the definitions? The definitions of reportable events vary among state laws, and there is little uniformity in terminology. For example, Colorado law refers to *occurrences,* Kansas law refers to *reportable incidents,* and Maine law refers to *sentinel events.* Definitions vary as much as the terminology. This makes it nearly impossible to aggregate or compare data across states, which is one of the IOM recommendations. In Pennsylvania, there are three types of reportable events: serious events, incidents, and infrastructure failures.

What agencies have enforcement authority? A state agency, such as a Department of Health, is usually responsible for promulgating detailed regulations that implement the state law, as well as for issuing periodic reports on the reporting system. Some states publish public reports in the form of, for example, aggregate facility-specific data, alerts, or newsletters (Leape, 2002). The Pennsylvania law establishes a new entity, the Patient Safety Authority. It is governed by an eleven-member board of directors and is responsible for managing the state's patient safety trust fund (funded by assessments on covered facilities). It is not a regulatory agency. As set forth in MCare, it has contracted with an independent entity to collect and analyze data regarding reports of serious events and incidents, issue recommendations for reducing serious events and incidents, receive and investigate anonymous reports, and report to state authorities on its activities.

What programs must covered facilities implement? In Pennsylvania, covered facilities must develop, implement, and comply with an internal patient safety plan. They are expected to consult with physicians, nurses, and other licensed providers when developing the internal patient safety plan, and to submit the plan to the Health Department for approval. Required elements of the plan include

- Designation of a patient safety officer
- Establishment of a patient safety committee
- Establishment of a round-the-clock system for health care workers to report serious events and near misses
- Prohibition of any retaliatory action against health care workers who report events or incidents
- Articulation of the process by which written notification of serious events will be provided to patients

What liaisons and committees are required? In Pennsylvania, each medical facility must designate a patient safety officer and create a patient safety committee. The patient safety officer will serve on the patient safety committee, ensure that serious events and incidents are investigated, report to the patient safety committee about actions to promote patient safety, and take action immediately when necessary to improve patient safety. The patient safety committee is to comprise at least three health care workers (including at least one nurse and one doctor), the patient safety officer, and two community residents who are not employed by the medical facility. Only one facility board member is allowed to be on the committee. The committee is responsible for

- Receiving reports from the patient safety officer.
- Evaluating investigations and actions of the patient safety officer as they relate to a report.
- Reviewing and evaluating the quality of patient safety measures.
- Making recommendations to eliminate future serious events or incidents.
- Reporting to the administrative officer and governing body of the medical facility on a quarterly basis; this report must include the number of serious events and incidents and recommendations to eliminate future serious events and incidents.

What reports must be submitted to the state? States often categorize types of reportable events. For example, they may use separate categories for serious injuries, deaths, sexual abuse cases, and near misses. Different categories often have different reporting requirements, such as the types of facilities that must submit reports, the state agency to which reports must be submitted, the time in which a report must be made, and the information that must accompany a report. The data that must be reported often include the name of the facility, type of incident, date of incident, description of incident, name of reporter, patient outcome, action taken by the facility, and root cause analysis results. Under the Pennsylvania law, health care workers who reasonably believe that a serious event or incident has occurred must report the event or incident through internal reporting channels as prescribed by the medical facility's patient safety plan. The report should be made immediately, or as soon as possible after the discovery of the event or incident, but no later than twenty-four hours after occurrence or discovery of the event or incident. There is a two-tiered external reporting system. Serious events or incidents must be reported to the state Health Department and the Patient Safety Authority. In addition, near misses must be reported to the Patient Safety Authority.

What are the penalties? In Pennsylvania, failure to report a serious event or infrastructure failure or to develop and comply with a patient safety plan as required by MCare constitutes a violation of state law. Failure to report a serious event or infrastructure failure or to notify a licensure board may result in an administrative penalty of $1,000 per day.

Are disclosures to patients required? A few states have passed legislation requiring that facilities report certain types of adverse events to patients or to their families. In Pennsylvania, written notification must be provided to patients affected by a serious event within seven days of the occurrence or discovery of the event. The law sets forth special circumstances under which family members should be notified and specifies that any such notifications shall not constitute an admission of liability.

What confidentiality protections are in place? There may be provisions that address the confidentiality of the reports. The Pennsylvania law includes confidentiality provisions that protect documents, materials, or information prepared or created pursuant to the responsibilities of the patient safety committee or governing board of the medical facility. Any documents, materials, and information prepared or created for the purposes of complying with the patient safety plan or with the reporting, notification, and investigation that are reviewed by the patient safety committee or governing board of the medical facility are confidential. They will not be discoverable or admissible as evidence in any civil or administrative action or proceeding. Persons responsible for or participating in meetings of the patient safety committee or governing board will not be required to testify about any matters within the knowledge gained because of a person's responsibilities or participation on the patient safety committee or governing board of the medical facility.

As of June 2004, more than 400 Pennsylvania facilities were reporting both actual events and near misses through the Pennsylvania Patient Safety Reporting System (PA-PSRS), a Web-based reporting system. The state has already begun to conduct analyses based on these reports, and it issues a quarterly newsletter, the *PA-PSRS Patient Safety Advisory*, with alerts and patient safety information.

Federal Patient Safety Legislation Initiatives

Many federal bills addressing voluntary reporting of adverse events were introduced in 2002 and 2003, and more are likely to be proposed in the years to come. Each offers a mechanism for protecting patient safety information from disclosure in litigation. For example, the Patient Safety Improvement Act of 2002 (HR 4889) would allow health care providers to report key patient safety data to a *patient safety organization* (PSO), which in turn would issue information on error prevention. The PSOs would deidentify information and then report it to the Department of Health and Human Services (HHS) Center for Quality Improvement and Patient Safety. The center would certify PSOs and maintain a database of patient safety information that could be used to identify national trends and prevent future errors. This proposed bill would prohibit the use of voluntary reports of medical errors as evidence in malpractice lawsuits, and grant confidentiality and peer review protections for medical error data provided under HHS safety improvement programs. The bill would direct the HHS secretary to establish mechanisms for analyzing aggregated, deidentified patient safety data to determine patterns of medical errors, to notify health care providers of steps they can take to reduce errors, and to analyze system changes adopted by providers and patient safety organizations in an effort to prevent future mistakes. It also calls for developing voluntary standards for the interoperability of health care information technology systems. This legislation would not interfere with the mandatory medical error reporting laws in twenty states.

The Patient Safety and Quality Improvement Act (S 2590) would make patient safety data privileged and confidential and therefore not subject to civil, criminal, or administrative proceedings unless a judge finds the release of the information meets a strong, three-pronged test: it must be (1) material to the proceeding, (2) within the public interest, and (3) not available from any other source. This bill would allow existing mandatory and voluntary reporting systems at the state level to be surveyed to identify their successes and failures. In addition, it would protect states' rights to maintain or create peer review and confidentiality protections that are stronger than what is required at the federal level.

The 108th Congress, as of early February 2003, had introduced several bills related to medical malpractice insurance and reform (see, for example, HR 321 introduced on January 8, 2003; HR 485 introduced on January 29, 2003; and HR 446 introduced January 29, 2003). The 109th Congress will likely face similar initiatives.

Medical Device Reporting

The concept of medical device reporting is not new. ECRI began its voluntary reporting program in 1971 and is still in operation, receiving reports of medical device adverse events and near misses from health care facilities, providers, and other sources.[4] ECRI's voluntary reporting system is independent, nonpunitive, and confidential. Reports are reviewed by experts who understand medical technology and its use and who provide timely feedback to reporters. As an independent, nonprofit agency, ECRI has no governmental authority to punish reporters, and thus reporting to it is viewed as safe. When ECRI identifies a device-related problem, it seeks an appropriate remedy from the medical device manufacturer, such as a design modification, repair, or replacement. In addition, ECRI issues *hazard reports*, with recommendations for preventing injury, and maintains the world's largest databases for medical device problems and hazards.

The medical device reporting (MDR) requirements of the Safe Medical Devices Act (SMDA) took effect on November 28, 1991. This Act requires user facilities to report certain adverse events involving medical devices to the device manufacturer and to the U.S. Food and Drug Administration (FDA). In December 1995, the FDA issued a final MDR rule that broadened the type of regulated facilities, required the use of specific reporting forms, and set various documentation and record-keeping requirements. (For comprehensive information on and tools for medical device reporting, see ECRI, 1996.) Medical device reporting, which applies to manufacturers as well as user facilities, is the FDA's version of an early warning system. It is intended to help the agency identify problems that pose a threat to health and safety. Under the rule, reports must be submitted whenever a user facility receives or otherwise becomes aware of information that reasonably suggests that a medical device has caused or may have caused or contributed to (a) the death of a patient or employee of the facility or (b) serious injury to a patient or employee of the user facility. Deaths must be reported to the medical device manufacturer and the FDA; serious injuries must be reported to the manufacturer. Both types of reports must be submitted within ten days of the facility's becoming aware of the information, using a special form (FDA Form 3500A). In addition to these ten-day individual event reports, user facilities must submit an annual report to FDA with information on all reports, both deaths and serious injuries, made during the previous calendar year (FDA Form 3419).

The FDA rule provides a broad definition of a user facility—hospitals, nursing homes, ambulatory surgical centers, outpatient treatment facilities, outpatient diagnostic facilities, home health agencies, blood banks, ambulance providers, rescue groups, skilled nursing facilities, psychiatric facilities, rehabilitation facilities, hospices, and all other outpatient treatment and diagnostic facilities other than physicians' offices. FDA also defines the term *serious injury,* and it is important for reporting institutions to study this definition because it signals when a report must be submitted. A *serious injury* is defined as an injury or illness that is (a) life threatening, (b) results in permanent impairment of a body function or permanent damage to a body structure, or (c) necessitates medical or surgical intervention to preclude permanent impairment of a body function or permanent damage to a body structure.

Manufacturers that receive ten-day reports from user facilities must obtain missing or incomplete information from the user report, and then submit the report to the FDA in accordance with time frames established by regulation.

User facilities are required to establish medical device reporting event files that contain the following: (a) information in the possession of the facility or references to information related to the adverse event, including all documentation of deliberations and decision-making processes used to determine whether an event was deemed reportable or not reportable, and (b) copies of all forms and other information related to the event submitted to the FDA or other entities. Event files must be maintained for two years from the date of the event.

As with other mandatory reporting schemes, there is concern about the confidentiality and protection of information collected and submitted as part of an investigation. SMDA provides statutory protections against the use of user facility reports in any civil action unless the user facility, individual, or physician who made the report had knowledge that the information in the report was false. However, the actual nature and scope of this protection is unclear, and user facilities have concerns about jeopardizing existing state peer review or other privileges that may protect deliberations involving a device-related adverse event.

Clinical Trials and Adverse-Event Reporting

Clinical trials have obvious patient safety ramifications for the human subject participants because the products or procedures being tested may pose harm as well as benefit. In recent years there has been increasing public attention to the patient safety aspects of clinical trials. The September 1999 death of eighteen-year-old gene therapy recipient Jesse Gelsinger prompted investigations by the National Institutes of Health (NIH) and the FDA. Investigators found that the researchers violated the trial's protocol, and the institution and the researchers were barred from conducting further clinical studies. Gelsinger's family sued the researchers and the clinical trial managers for damages. In ensuing investigations, the FDA and NIH found that the researchers and institutions had failed to report adverse events although required by regulation to do.

Adverse-event reporting is a critical element of the regulatory system and is covered by both HHS and FDA regulations. The goals are in alignment with the patient safety movement in that reporting is intended to prompt investigation and evaluation of causes and corrective actions and dissemination of this knowledge to researchers in other trials so they will take appropriate steps to protect their subjects. HHS requires institutional review boards (IRBs) to have written procedures for ensuring "prompt reporting" to the IRB, appropriate institutional officials, and the relevant department or agency head of any unanticipated problems involving risks to subjects or others or any serious or continuing noncompliance issues. FDA regulations for investigational new drug applications require the sponsor to report an adverse experience in writing to the FDA and all participating investigators within fifteen calendar days if the event is both serious and unexpected and by telephone or facsimile within seven calendar days if it is life threatening or fatal. All other adverse experiences and outcomes must be summarized in the annual report to the FDA and the IRB.

These rules are based on the commonsense notion that those who manage new technologies, the risks of which are yet unknown, should learn to make improvements in safety on a continuing basis. They should capture experiential information on harmful incidents immediately, determine their root causes and contributing factors, and take corrective action to prevent recurrence of the incidents, including but not limited to disclosure.

Patient Safety Goals and Standards

In July 2002, the JCAHO board of commissioners approved the 2003 National Patient Safety Goals (NPSGs). New goals and recommendations are announced each July and become effective on January 1 of the following year. JCAHO-accredited health care organizations are surveyed for implementation of the goals and recommendations, as part of either a scheduled survey or a random unannounced survey. Under the JCAHO revised survey process, when an accredited facility receives a *requirement of improvement* for noncompliance with an NPSG, that issue must be addressed in the *evidence for standards compliance* (ESC) report. This report must include evidence of actions taken to achieve compliance with all NPSG requirements. If an accredited organization fails to demonstrate full compliance, its accreditation status will be changed to provisional accreditation. There is a formal process for seeking JCAHO approval of an alternate approach. The 2004 goals are as follows (JCAHO, 2004):

1. Improve the accuracy of patient identification.
   a. Use at least two patient identifiers (neither to be the patient's room number) whenever taking blood samples or administering medications or blood products.
   b. Prior to the start of any surgical or invasive procedure, conduct a final verification process, such as a "time out," to confirm the correct patient, procedure and site, using active—not passive—communication techniques.
2. Improve the effectiveness of communication among caregivers.
   a. Implement a process for taking verbal or telephone orders . . . that require a verification "read-back" of the complete order . . . by the person receiving the order . . .
   b. Standardize the abbreviations, acronyms and symbols used throughout the organization, including a list of abbreviations, acronyms and symbols *not* to use.
3. Improve the safety of using high-alert medications.
   a. Remove concentrated electrolytes (including, but not limited to, potassium chloride, potassium phosphate, sodium chloride >0.9%) from patient care units.
   b. Standardize and limit the number of drug concentrations available in the organization.

4. Eliminate wrong-site, wrong-patient, wrong-procedure surgery.
   a. Create and use a preoperative verification process, such as a checklist, to confirm that appropriate documents (e.g., medical records, imaging studies) are available.
   b. Implement a process to mark the surgical . . . site and involve the patient in the marking process.
5. Improve the safety of using infusion pumps.
   a. Ensure free-flow protection on all general-use and PCA (patient controlled analgesia) intravenous infusion pumps used in the organization.
6. Improve the effectiveness of clinical alarm systems.
   a. Implement regular preventive maintenance and testing of alarm systems.
   b. Assure that alarms are activated with appropriate settings and are sufficiently audible with respect to distances and competing noise within the unit.
7. Reduce the risk of health care–acquired infections.
   a. Comply with current CDC hand hygiene guidelines.
   b. Manage as sentinel events all identified cases of unanticipated death or major permanent loss of function associated with a health care–acquired infection.

For 2005, JCAHO developed program-specific goals for all accreditation programs, such as ambulatory, assisted living, behavioral health care, critical access hospital, disease-specific care, home care, hospital, laboratory, long-term care, and office-based surgery. New goals include reconciliation of medication across the continuum of care and reduction of the risk of patient falls, of contracting influenza, and of surgical fires.[5]

The NPSGs are derived from a pool of recommendations previously issued by JCAHO in its *Sentinel Event Alert* newsletters as well as input from JCAHO committees, literature review, and other relevant databases.[6] The goals, along with their associated requirements, are selected by a JCAHO advisory group. Each year, new recommendations from the *Sentinel Event Alerts* published in the previous year and from other relevant sources are added to the pool and the advisory group reevaluates the goals and recommendations and recommends modifications, additions, or deletions for the next year. The advisory group's recommendations for annual NPSGs and associated recommendations are forwarded to JCAHO's board of commissioners for approval prior to the year in which they are to be implemented.

Although the NPSGs are not laws or mandatory regulations, they may nevertheless have legal value and consequence for a health care facility or provider being sued for medical malpractice. The introduction of safe practice standards into medical malpractice litigation is not new. The standards developed by medical specialty societies, such as the American Society of Anesthesiologists (ASA) and the American College of Obstetricians and Gynecologists (ACOG), have been introduced in court as evidence for over two decades. So have JCAHO standards. They have been used to help establish the applicable standard of care, which must be defined in each medical malpractice case. The medical profession itself, through expert testimony, sets the standard of care in most cases. Nonetheless, certain authoritative patient safety standards may provide a definition of the standard of care in certain cases and thus are of interest to medical malpractice litigants. A claimant in a malpractice case has the burden of proving that he or she was injured by care or treatment that failed to reach the standard of care reasonably expected of the medical practitioner. It would follow therefore that a physician or a hospital that complied with the patient safety standard could have a very good defense in a malpractice case: that is, a physician could use the standard or recommendation as a shield. Conversely, failure to comply could be used as evidence of negligence in a malpractice case: that is, the claimant could use the guidelines as a sword.

Key questions are whether a standard will be admitted into evidence and, if so, what weight it will be accorded. It may be necessary to qualify the standard as one that is in fact authoritative and has properly qualified authors, much in the way that an expert witness must be qualified to render an opinion. Some courts require an expert to testify as to the authority of the specific standard or guideline; others are willing to admit clinical practice guidelines as evidence without expert testimony. A 1993 U.S. Supreme Court decision (*Daubert* v. *Merrell Dow Pharmaceuticals*) created stricter standards for the judicial evaluation of the reliability and authoritativeness of proffered scientific evidence. That decision may encourage judges to scrutinize the process by which a standard was developed as well as the credentials and motivations of the issuing organization. The rules of admissibility are still being tested.

In any event, it is worth noting that compliance with a standard or recommendation may not necessarily be exculpatory because a jury might find that conduct above and beyond that standard was needed in order to meet the applicable standard of care.

The Quality Assessment and Performance Improvement Rule

On January 23, 2003, the Centers for Medicare & Medicaid Services published a new rule instructing hospitals to develop and implement quality improvement programs in an effort to further reduce medical errors (42 *C.F.R.* § 482.21, 2003).

This rule revised the quality assurance condition of participation (CoP) for hospitals that was issued in 1986.

Under the quality assessment and performance improvement (QAPI) rule, hospitals must develop, implement, and maintain an effective, ongoing, hospital-wide, data-driven QAPI program. The hospital's governing body must ensure that the program reflects the complexity of the hospital's organization and services, involves all hospital departments and services (including those services furnished under contract or arrangement), and focuses on indicators related to improved health outcomes and the prevention and reduction of medical errors. In defining the term *medical error,* CMS adopted the definition used by the Quality Interagency Coordination (QuIC) Task Force: "the failure of a planned action to be completed as intended or the use of a wrong plan to achieve an aim" (Quality Interagency Coordination Task Force, 2000). Errors may include problems with practices, products, procedures, and systems. The hospital must maintain and demonstrate evidence of its QAPI program for review by CMS.

There are five standards in the QAPI rule:

1. *Program scope.* The rule requires an ongoing program that shows measurable improvement in indicators for which there is evidence that they will improve outcomes. Hospitals must measure, analyze, and track quality indicators including adverse patient events.
2. *Program data.* The rule requires hospitals to use quality indicator data to monitor the effectiveness of services and identify opportunities for improvement.
3. *Program activities.* The rule requires hospitals to set priorities for performance improvement activities that focus on high-risk, high-volume, or problem-prone areas; consider the incidence, prevalence, and severity of problems in those areas; and affect health outcomes, patient safety, and quality of care. Performance improvement activities must track medical errors and adverse patient events, analyze their causes, and implement preventive actions and mechanisms that include feedback and learning throughout the hospital.
4. *Performance improvement projects.* The rule requires hospitals to conduct performance improvement projects of a number and scope proportional to the scope and complexity of the hospital's services and operations. One of these projects may be the development of an information technology system explicitly designed to improve patient safety and quality of care, and such a project, in its initial stage of development, does not need to demonstrate measurable improvement in indicators related to health outcome.
5. *Executive responsibilities.* The rule requires that the hospital's governing body, medical staff, and administrative officials are responsible and accountable for ensuring the following: (1) that an ongoing program for quality improvement

and patient safety, including the reduction of medical errors, is defined, implemented, and maintained; (2) that the hospital-wide quality assessment and performance improvement efforts address priorities for improved quality of care and patient safety and that all improvement actions are evaluated; (3) that clear expectations for safety are established; (4) that adequate resources are allocated for measuring, assessing, improving, and sustaining the hospital's performance and reducing risk to patients; and (5) that the determination of the number of distinct improvement projects is conducted annually.

If the state agency surveyors, following the existing survey process and procedures, determine that a hospital is significantly out of compliance with the QAPI CoP requirements, the hospital is scheduled for termination from the Medicare and Medicaid programs. The hospital then is given the opportunity to submit a plan of correction. Prior to the termination, the state agency conducts a follow-up survey to assess whether the hospital is now in compliance with all the requirements.

Smallpox Vaccine Adverse-Event Reporting

Bioterrorism and the Homeland Security Act of 2002 are likely to engender yet more adverse-event reporting and safety requirements for patients, health care workers, and the general population. In February 2003, the Centers for Disease Control and Prevention (CDC) announced the Smallpox Vaccine Adverse Events Monitoring and Response System ("Smallpox Vaccine . . . ," 2003) to deal with adverse reactions to smallpox vaccination. Information from this system will be regularly communicated to vaccine safety oversight groups, public health and medical communities, and the media. This system will be used (1) to monitor the occurrence of known adverse events after vaccination and to identify new and unexpected adverse events, (2) to monitor the effectiveness of screening for contraindications to vaccination, (3) to identify new contraindications that may emerge, and (4) to coordinate the distribution of Vaccinia Immune Globulin (VIG) and cidofovir, if these medications are needed for treatment of patients with certain severe adverse events.

Conclusion

Federal and state laws as well as accreditation requirements will continue to shape the landscape of patient safety. Many of the new statutes and regulations are apt to set minimal thresholds for patient safety. Others may be more exacting, requiring health care organizations to engage in a greater degree of reporting with a view to gathering data useful for patient safety.

Other laws may set standards or requirements for patient safety. Rather than focusing on data aggregation, these requirements will set the norms for expected performance levels.

As the law evolves in this arena, it is essential that health care organizations keep abreast of changes at the federal and state levels. Such attention to detail will be imperative for compliance with patient safety expectations and legal requirements.

Notes

1. Patient safety laws and regulations are not limited to the United States. The United Kingdom's National Health Service has established the National Patient Safety Agency, which is tasked with operating and enforcing a national mandatory reporting system for adverse events. Japan has launched a national patient safety effort. In 2002, the World Health Organization (WHO) adopted a resolution making patient safety a high priority for its policy agenda, and it has begun to focus on developing nations (WHO, 2003).
2. These states are California, Colorado, Connecticut, Florida, Georgia, Kansas, Maine, Maryland, Massachusetts, Minnesota, New Jersey, New York, Nevada, Ohio, Pennsylvania, Rhode Island, South Carolina, South Dakota, Tennessee, Texas, Utah, Washington.
3. The Pennsylvania Patient Safety Authority selected ECRI as the contractor to develop and implement the reporting system in partnership with ISMP and EDS (http://www.psa.state.pa.us/psa/lib/psa/press_releases/ecri-_press_release_vers_4___7-31-03.pdf).
4. ECRI (http://www.ecri.org) is an independent, nonprofit research agency located in Plymouth Meeting, Pennsylvania, with numerous programs in health care risk management, patient safety, evidence-based technology assessment, and medical device safety. For information on medical device safety alerts, see http://www.mdsr.ecri.org.
5. For updates to the NPSGs, see JCAHO's Web site at http://www.jcaho.org/accredited+organizations/patient+safety/npsg.htm.
6. *Sentinel Event Alerts* are published as necessary by JCAHO and are available on the JCAHO Web site at http://www.jcaho.org.

References

Daubert v. *Merrell Dow Pharmaceuticals, Inc.,* 509 U.S. 579 (1993).

ECRI. *Final Report: Medical Device Reporting Under the Safe Medical Devices Act.* Plymouth Meeting, Penn.: ECRI, 1996.

Institute of Medicine. *Crossing the Quality Chasm: A New Health System for the 21st Century.* Washington, D.C.: National Academies Press, 2001.

Institute of Medicine. *Patient Safety: Achieving a New Standard for Care.* Washington, D.C.: National Academies Press, 2004.

Joint Commission on Accreditation of Healthcare Organizations. "2004 National Patient Safety Goals."
[http://www.jcaho.org/accredited+organizations/patient+safety/npsg.htm]. 2004.

Kohn, L. T., Corrigan, J. M., and Donaldson, M. S. (eds.). *To Err Is Human: Building a Safer Health System.* Washington, D.C.: National Academies Press, 2000.

Leape, L. "Reporting of Adverse Events." *New England Journal of Medicine,* Nov. 14, 2002, *347,* 1633–1638.

National Academy for State Health Policy. "Quality and Patient Safety." [http://www.nashp.org/_docdisp_page.cfm?LID=2A789909-5310-11D6-BCF000A0CC558925]. Mar. 2004.

O'Connell, J., and Bryan, P. "More Hippocrates, Less Hypocrisy: 'Early Offers' as a Means of Implementing the Institute of Medicine's Recommendations on Malpractice Law." *Journal of Law and Health,* Mar. 2000, *15,* 23–51.

Pennsylvania Patient Safety Authority. *PA-PSRS Patient Safety Advisory.* Newsletter. [http://www.psa.state.pa.us]. Various dates.

Quality Interagency Coordination Task Force. *Doing What Counts for Patient Safety: Federal Actions to Reduce Medical Errors and Their Impact.* Publication No. OM 00-0004. Rockville, Md.: Agency for Healthcare Research and Quality, Feb. 2000.

Reardon, T. R. Statement of the American Medical Association to the Subcommittee of Health, Committee on Ways and Means, U.S. House of Representatives, Feb. 10, 2000.

Rosenthal, J., Booth, M., Flowers, L., and Riley T. *Current State Programs Addressing Medical Errors: An Analysis of Mandatory Reporting and Other Initiatives.* Portland, Maine: National Academy for State Health Policy, Jan. 2001.

"Smallpox Vaccine Adverse Events Monitoring and Response System for the First State of the Smallpox Vaccination Program." *Morbidity and Mortality Weekly Report.* [http://www.cdc.gov/od/oc/media/mmwrnews/n030207.htm]. Feb. 7, 2003.

Studdert, D., and Brennan, T. "No-Fault Compensation for Medical Injuries: The Prospect for Error Prevention." *Journal of the American Medical Association,* July 11, 2001, *286,* 217–223.

World Health Organization. *Patient Safety: Rapid Assessment Methods for Estimating Hazards.* Report of the WHO Working Group Meeting. Geneva: World Health Organization, Jan. 2003.

CHAPTER THREE

MEDICAL ERROR REDUCTION INITIATIVES AMONG ACCREDITATION AND STANDARD-SETTING ORGANIZATIONS

Fay A. Rozovsky

Many believe it was the publication of the Institute of Medicine (IOM) report *To Err Is Human* (Kohn, Corrigan, and Donaldson, 2000) that drove the focused interest in patient safety of the Joint Commission on Accreditation of Healthcare Organizations (JCAHO). In fact the Joint Commission's interest predated the IOM report. One could argue that the entire JCAHO accreditation process, dating back to its inception in 1952, has been focused on patient safety. Although not labeled as such, the idea of an outside organization measuring health care institution performance against a set of quality-based standards is about enhancing the opportunities for patient safety.

The Joint Commission joined the fight for patient safety in a more formal way with its efforts in the 1990s to address sentinel events. The Joint Commission was, however, not the only accrediting body interested in this topic. Once again, although not addressing their work in terms of patient safety, the efforts of other well-recognized accrediting organizations shared the same idea of promoting quality patient care. A review of the work product of the National Committee for Quality Assurance (NCQA), the Commission on Accreditation of Rehabilitation Facilities (CARF), the Community Health Accreditation Program (CHAP), and the Healthcare Facilities Accreditation Program (HFAP) of the American Osteopathic Association (AOA), among others, demonstrates a shared commitment to the ideals of patient safety. Indeed, in many ways the terms *quality* and *risk management* have been operative phrases for creating an environment of care that is safe for patients, their loved ones, and staff.

Accreditation organizations are not the only sources for private sector standards devoted to patient safety. Rather than follow the deemed agency model, in which the requirements of the standards organization are surrogates for the Conditions of Participation in Medicare and Medicaid, other private sector groups have developed their own norms for achieving what they envisage patient safety to be. Among these groups are the National Quality Forum (NQF) and the Leapfrog Group.

Issue-specific safety concerns have long been the focal point of yet other organizations. For example, the National Fire Protection Association (NFPA) has set the norms for *life safety* in health care facilities. Similarly, APIC, the Association for Professionals in Infection Control and Epidemiology, has had a focused interest in infection control, and many of the prominent specialty colleges in medicine have established norms for their respective areas of practice. Sometimes these norms are phrased as guidelines, statements, or position statements (see, for example, the "Basic Standards for Preanesthesia Care" of the American Society of Anesthesiologists, 1987). However characterized, the statements of these groups are geared to quality, safe patient care.

Yet another avenue to medical error reduction has been to incorporate the International Organization for Standardization (ISO) approach and also Six Sigma methods into the health care field. The ISO has long been known in industry for its standard-setting approach to continuous quality improvement. This approach has now made its way into the health care arena in Australia, New Zealand, and the United Kingdom. It also has met with limited success in the United States. Six Sigma, a methodology with a set of sophisticated quality tools used in industry, is slowly garnering attention in the health care field. The idea is to use these statistical tools to achieve and maintain a certain norm—six sigma—in terms of quality and medical error.

What are not addressed in many quarters are the legal and regulatory aspects of these private sector initiatives in patient safety. Some key questions need to be examined. For example, do these private sector standards set a higher duty of care than that required by federal or state regulations? From the regulatory point of view, what should be the consequence for a health care organization that is noncompliant with a group of private sector medical error reduction initiatives? These topics are addressed in this chapter. Rather than discouraging a health care facility from embracing private sector patient safety initiatives, the idea is to develop a framework of ways health care organizations can use these standards without subjecting themselves to unwanted and unanticipated litigation.

JCAHO Patient Safety Initiatives

Patient safety and medical error reduction have been part of the fabric of JCAHO for many years. As suggested earlier, it can be argued that patient safety has been a focal point since the organization's inception. Like other national accrediting bodies, JCAHO enjoys *deemed status* under federal regulatory requirements. In essence this means that the standards followed by JCAHO and its process of accreditation serve as a vehicle for obtaining certification under the Conditions of Participation (CoPs) in Medicare and Medicaid. The Centers for Medicare & Medicaid Services (CMS) have established different CoPs for each type of health care facility. In the case of hospitals the CoPs speak specifically to patient safety (64 *Fed. Reg.* 127, 36069–36089, July 2, 1999).

For accredited healthcare organizations, there is a two-for-one benefit. Not only does the entity receive accreditation status, it also receives certification for Medicare and Medicaid. Thus accreditation eliminates the need for a state agency to perform a survey to ascertain if the facility should receive certification under the CoPs for Medicare and Medicaid. It often is suggested that this one-step process saves considerable time and money. However, it does not preclude a state agency from performing a validation survey, a process designed to confirm that the health care facility is in fact in compliance with the Conditions of Participation. Successfully completing the JCAHO accreditation process also enhances the accredited organization's opportunity to become a designated residency training facility.

Patient Safety Standards

JCAHO standards are not a mirror image of the Conditions of Participation for any type of health care organization. In the case of hospitals, for example, the JCAHO requirements exceed the CoPs. This is seen in the area of patient safety. In 2001, JCAHO put into effect a new set of patient safety standards for accredited hospitals. Included in these standards were requirements with respect to establishing patient safety standards, developing a culture of safety under the direction of hospital leadership, using prospective analytical tools to prevent medical errors (including medication errors), redesigning processes for patient safety, and disclosing outcomes of care to patients (JCAHO, 2004a). In January 2003, patient safety standards for behavioral and long-term care facilities were put into effect, and in January 2004, the patient safety standards for home care ambulatory care organizations were put into effect.

Staffing Effectiveness

JCAHO has taken a particular interest in staffing effectiveness with respect to patient care. Certain types of indicators have been built into the accreditation process in the hope that these data will identify opportunities for improvement related to patient safety. Other entities have manifested a similar concern about the relationship of staffing ratios to patient safety. Indeed, California has established statutory requirements for staff-patient ratios (California Business & Professions Act § 2725.3, effective 2004; *California Health Safety Code* § 1276.4, effective 2004).

Further information is needed to determine the extent to which *types* of staffing make a difference in patient safety. For example, is it merely the number of nurses per patient or is it the number of specialty-trained nurses per patient that makes a difference? Is it the nurse-patient ratio or is it the number of continuous hours of nursing service provided by a professional that makes a difference? As more information becomes available in this area, perhaps some clarity will begin to emerge about what truly is important to patient safety when one is setting professional staffing ratios.

Sentinel Event Policy

In 1996, JCAHO implemented a *sentinel event* policy. The idea was to identify, report, evaluate, and prevent sentinel events. Conducting root cause analysis of such events, health care organizations use the resulting information to conduct process redesign with a view to preventing the occurrence of similar events in the future. Monitoring the effectiveness of the change in the process also is part of the sentinel event policy.

JCAHO wanted health care organizations to share their results with JCAHO in the hope that the aggregated information would point the way toward needed advances in medical error reduction. The *Sentinel Event Alerts* published by JCAHO are a reflection of the collective information received in the key areas defined in the sentinel event policy. For JCAHO the sentinel event policy is a key ingredient of the patient safety standards and of the overall effort toward medical error reduction.

Patient Safety Goals

In 2002, JCAHO launched its first set of National Patient Safety Goals (for the 2004 goals, see JCAHO, 2004b). Each health care facility's performance with respect to the goals is reviewed during the on-site accreditation survey. Each goal has one or two evidence-based or expert-based recommendations. It is expected that *all* the goals will be met by an accredited organization. The goals are recommended by a multidisciplinary advisory group. Each year the group reviews the content to determine whether some goals should be deleted and whether new ones should be added as priority safety practice areas. Accredited organizations also may suggest goals for review by the advisory group.

The Periodic Performance Report

Greater emphasis on continuous operational improvement is at the forefront of JCAHO's Shared Visions—New Pathways approach to accreditation ("The Launch of Shared Visions—New Pathways," 2004). This approach encompasses a review midway through the accreditation process to ascertain whether the organization is compliant with standards. Evaluation is premised on the standards and the *elements of performance* (EPs) found with each standard. A *priority focus process* (PFP) also is applied during accreditation, using information specific to the health care organization to identify the top four clinical service group areas and priority focus areas for that facility.

In response to some legal concerns involving evidentiary protection of *periodic performance report* (PPR) information placed on the JCAHO extranet, JCAHO created some nonextranet options: completion of a self-assessment of compliance with the standards (PPR Option 1); an on-site survey by JCAHO, with the organization providing a plan of action for noncompliant areas within thirty days (PPR Option 2); and an on-site, midcycle survey by JCAHO in which the surveyor leaves behind no written report and provides findings verbally to the organization (PPR Option 3).

Quality Reports

The Shared Visions—New Pathways reformation of the accreditation process establishes a new way for the Joint Commission to display its findings. The idea is to make the process more understandable to users of the information. JCAHO *quality reports* present information on compliance with the National Patient Safety Goals and the National Quality Improvement Goals and also benchmark comparisons with other JCAHO accredited hospitals. The reports also encompass "patient experience of care" information. The findings for each accredited hospital are published under the "Quality Check" component of the JCAHO Web site.

Patient Safety in Other Accreditation Standards

Patient safety is of concern to other accrediting organizations. Like JCAHO, they emphasize quality and safety. For example, in the Managed Behavioral Healthcare Organization (MBHO) Accreditation Program of the National

Committee for Quality Assurance (NCQA), specific standards address patient safety. Chapter Twelve of the Healthcare Facilities Accreditation Program (HFAP) of the American Osteopathic Association (AOA) tracks the quality assessment and performance improvement (QAPI) regulation promulgated by the CMS (68 *Fed. Reg.* 16, 3435–3455, Jan. 24, 2003). This regulation addresses the leadership responsibilities for quality care and patient safety. Thus the HFAP accreditation program has incorporated the federal parameters for patient safety.

Whether mentioned as a stand-alone element or included in the broader picture of quality of care, patient safety is an issue of concern for all accreditation bodies. Hospitals are not the only targets for such activity. To the extent that the topic is addressed in accreditation standards, it is a reflection of widespread concern that all types of health care entities meet a minimum level of service that promotes quality and patient safety.

The Leapfrog Group and the NQF as Standard-Setting Organizations

Two groups have emerged as key standard-setting organizations. Neither group is engaged in accreditation. One, the Leapfrog Group, comprises some 150 public and private organizations that provide health care benefits. It identifies problems and possible solutions for improving hospital systems. After examining scientific information, the Leapfrog Group chose computerized physician order entry (CPOE); evidence-based hospital referral (EHR), sometimes known as high-volume referral; and ICU physician staffing (IPS) as activities that would likely help save lives by reducing preventable mistakes occurring in hospitals.

The National Quality Forum (NQF) is a not-for-profit membership organization whose stated mission is "to improve American healthcare through endorsement of consensus-based national standards for measurement and public reporting of healthcare performance data that provide meaningful information about whether care is safe, timely, beneficial, patient-centered, equitable and efficient" (NQF, 2004). In 2003, NQF issued a report titled *Safe Practices for Better Healthcare: A Consensus Report* that set forth thirty *safe practices* that NQF believed would reduce the risk of injury in the health care field. The thirty safe practices were divided into these five broad categories (p. vi):

Creating a culture of safety;

Matching healthcare needs with service delivery capability;

Facilitating information transfer and clear communication;

Adopting safe practices in specific clinical care settings or for specific processes of care; and,

Increasing safe medication use.

In April 2004, the Leapfrog Group adopted the NQF safe practices as its fourth area of focus. The NQF adopted the three areas of CPOE, HER, and IPS set forth by the Leapfrog Group.

Taken together the Leapfrog and NQF initiatives demonstrate private sector efforts to create patient safety standards. NQF's safe practices now have been codified into law in two states (see *Minnesota Statutes* §§ 144.706–144.7069, 2003; Connecticut Public Act No. 04-164, effective July 1, 2004). This reflects the fact that state legislators, concerned about patient safety, will reach out for initiatives that they believe will help reduce the risk of patient injury in the health care setting.

Environment of Care Safety

Historically, JCAHO and other accrediting bodies have focused on the *environment of care.* Safety and security have been focal points of accreditation standards. Other organizations also have been involved in this area. Notable among them is the National Fire Protection Association (NFPA). *Standards for Health Care Facilities* (NFPA, 1999, 2002) covers a host of environment of care items, such as environmental systems, electrical systems, gas and vacuum systems, electrical equipment, gas equipment, and manufacturer requirements.

The National Fire Protection Association requirements for health care represent just one set of standards from this organization. In the broader context, NFPA is responsible for over 300 consensus codes and standards, including the Life Safety Code (NFPA, 2003) that is applicable to health care facilities. The NFPA dates back to 1896. An international nonprofit organization, its stated mission is "to reduce the worldwide burden of fire and other hazards on the quality of life by providing and advocating scientifically-based consensus codes and standards, research, training and education" (NFPA, 2004). Like other nonaccrediting organizations, NFPA has a well-respected and well-recognized role in setting standards for safety.

ISO and Six Sigma

The International Organization for Standardization, or ISO, comprises national standards institutes from 148 countries. A central secretariat in Geneva, Switzerland, coordinates the system. Although it is a nongovernmental organization, many of its member institutes are part of the governmental structure in their respective countries. Other members are mandated by their national governments. Still other members have emerged from the private sector as established industry associations.

The ISO develops standards when there is an identified market need. Thus far the ISO has produced more than 13,700 international standards. Two categories, ISO 9000 and ISO 14000, are generic, providing a framework on which those who use the standards can fill in the detail for specific industries. This has been accomplished for the health care arena with respect to health care risk management. This standard is different from others published by ISO that address different aspects of the health care field, such as equipment standardization or sterilization.

Standards Australia first published "Guidelines for Managing Risk in the Healthcare Sector." These guidelines have since been embraced by standards organizations in other countries, including Standards New Zealand. The content is premised on ISO 9000 and its generic template. In it, Standards Australia establishes a framework for risk management in the health care field, with content for board members and senior management personnel as well as clinical staff.

In the context of creating a culture of safety and at the same time meeting the CMS regulatory requirements for quality assessment and performance improvement, the ISO provisions may serve as a useful framework. At the very least the ISO specific standards shed light on another approach to standard setting with the goal of reducing the risk of patient injury in the health care field.

Six Sigma, as mentioned earlier, is a methodology and a set of sophisticated quality tools used in industry to reduce process variation. Six Sigma tools include root cause analysis, failure modes and effects analysis, statistical process controls, run charts, and control charts. Projects are selected for application of the Six Sigma tools. Individuals—black belts and green belts—who have received special training in the use of Six Sigma tools and in guiding the projects assist in the work activity. Interestingly, many of the tools in the Six Sigma tool chest have found their way into the health care field thanks to the patient safety efforts of JCAHO. Root cause analysis, failure modes and effects analysis, and statistical process controls are found in the current set of accreditation standards. However, the JCAHO standards do not incorporate the degree of detail in use in Six Sigma consulting practices or in trade associations such as the American Society for Quality (ASQ).

Whether Six Sigma will receive widespread acceptance as a patient safety tool is still uncertain. There are some observers in the health care field who see Six Sigma as nothing more than an expensive, time-consuming next step in the quality movement. In a field strapped for funding and personnel to meet its fundamental obligations to patient care, there are those who think Six Sigma is better applied in industry—not health care.

Clinical Practice Guidelines

Guidelines, protocols, clinical pathways, and position statements have received widespread attention as the health care field has moved to evidence-based research to substantiate the validity of such norms. Rather than relying on anecdotal information, or expert experience alone, the health care field has sought a scientific basis for deciding what norms to follow in the delivery of care. To the extent that these norms prevent injury and enhance patient safety, they may be recognized as standards of care.

Many national organizations have developed guidelines relating to health care, and many of these sets of guidelines have been collected by the National Guideline Clearinghouse, which is an initiative of the Agency for Healthcare Research and Quality (AHRQ, 2004). Looked at in their entirety, these guidelines reflect a common desire to develop practical approaches to reducing the risk of patient injury in health care. Created in nongovernmental settings, the guidelines demonstrate that national groups can serve as incubators of clinically appropriate practices for patient safety.

The Legal and Regulatory Consequences of Private Sector Patient Safety Initiatives

As discussed in Chapter One, establishing a standard should be considered carefully in light of the financial, material, and personnel requirements associated with implementation. In addition to those requirements found in statutes and regulations, a health care organization imposes voluntary standards upon itself. This means that health care leaders can exercise considerable judgment as to the utility, value, and significance of one set of standards as compared to another.

Standards selection should not be taken lightly. Once adopted, standards can have significant legal consequences. A failure to meet a self-imposed or voluntarily adopted standard that results in reasonably foreseeable harm or injury may serve as the context for negligence litigation. In the contractual setting the failure to meet standards may lead to allegations of a breach culminating in the termination of the agreement. If the contract was with a health plan, the termination of the agreement may mean considerable loss in revenue.

Following accreditation standards, a voluntary process for health care organizations, also can have legal repercussions. Regulators may react, especially if an accrediting body finds standards noncompliance that leads to an "immediate threat to life" finding. When a deemed agency makes a determination of serious noncompliance that raises the specter of possible immediate harm to patients, federal regulators and state agencies may start the process that can culminate in decertification for purposes of Medicare and Medicaid reimbursement.

Nevertheless, the potential for legal repercussions should not deter health care organizations from embracing standards or the accreditation process. Rather, knowing that there are legal concerns, health care organizations can approach standards adaptation wisely in the area of patient safety. Some helpful strategies include the following:

- Provide the requisite financial, material, and personnel resources essential for patient safety.
- Ensure that leadership exerts itself in setting the norm for a culture of safety.
- Provide practical educational opportunities for all personnel to learn how to apply the standards.
- Establish effective communication systems to support standards adaptation, design, and implementation.
- Implement a system for measuring performance and the utility of the standards adopted.
- Implement a system for ongoing standards improvement that incorporates relevant data.
- Encourage professionals to challenge standards that appear inappropriate or a threat to patient safety, and provide a process for standards exception when there is a risk of patient injury.
- Anticipate key concerns that may come to light as a consequence of standard adaptation and standard noncompliance (when, for example, private sector standards require a higher duty of care than that required by federal or state regulations), and consider the fallout if the health care organization is noncompliant with a group of private sector medical error reduction initiatives.

Conclusion

Standards are an important factor in medical error reduction, enhanced patient safety, and quality care. Standards emanate from many sources, both governmental and nongovernmental. Weaving together the right set of standards requires leadership and effective relationships between management and professionals in health care organizations. It is a challenge that must be met for the well-being of patient care.

References

Agency for Healthcare Research and Quality, National Guideline Clearinghouse. [http://www.guideline.gov]. 2004.

American Society of Anesthesiologists. "Basic Standards for Preanesthesia Care." Park Ridge, Ill.: American Society for Anesthesiologists, 1987. (Affirmed in 1998.)

Joint Commission on Accreditation of Healthcare Organizations. *Setting the Standard: The Joint Commission & Health Care Safety and Quality.* Oakbrook Terrace, Ill.: Joint Commission on Accreditation of Healthcare Organizations, 2004a.

Joint Commission on Accreditation of Healthcare Organizations. "2004 National Patient Safety Goals." [http://www.jcaho.org/accredited+organizations/patient+safety/npsg.htm]. 2004b.

Kohn, L. T., Corrigan, J. M., and Donaldson M. S. (eds.). *To Err Is Human: Building a Safer Health System.* Washington, D.C.: National Academies Press, 2000.

"The Launch of Shared Visions—New Pathways." *Joint Commission Perspectives,* Jan. 2004, *24*(1, entire issue).

National Fire Protection Association. *Standards for Health Care Facilities.* Quincy, Mass.: National Fire Protection Association, 1999, 2002.

National Fire Protection Association. "Life Safety Code." Quincy, Mass.: National Fire Protection Association, 2003.

National Fire Protection Association. "About NFPA." [http://www.nfpa.org/catalog/home/AboutNFPA/index.asp]. 2004.

National Quality Forum. *Safe Practices for Better Healthcare: A Consensus Report.* NQF-CR-05-03. Washington, D.C.: National Quality Forum, 2003.

National Quality Forum. "Mission." [http://www.qualityforum.org/mission/home.htm]. 2004.

CHAPTER FOUR

FAILURE MODES AND EFFECTS ANALYSIS

The Risks and the Rewards in Health Care

Robert J. Latino

Failure modes and effects analysis . . . what a complex sounding and intimidating name! Although the FMEA methodology has been around for decades, it is relatively new to the health care world. The very name itself, failure modes and effects analysis, suggests that engineers had a hand in its original development. Engineers, known for their left-brain tendencies, are stereotyped as logical individuals who plan and structure everything. Seen through an engineer's eyes, the world is a complex system in which the known sciences must apply to solve all problems.

Contrast this to what engineers are not characteristically known for—that is their right-brain tendencies or the ability to be creative and think in the abstract or in concepts (versus the definitiveness of known science). Herein lies the crossroads at which FMEA meets health care. Recent efforts by the Joint Commission on Accreditation of Healthcare Organizations (JCAHO) attempt to utilize FMEA and apply it to health care systems. This is an admirable effort and, this author believes, a well-founded one. However, the cultural differences between industry and health care must be taken into consideration and accounted for in order for this initiative to be successful.

Traditional FMEA Roots

Start with an understanding of the original intent of FMEA. It is a foundation for determining what modifications would be appropriate for FMEA in the health care environment. Consider that the FMEA technique was born in the aircraft industry, and FMEA is most widely known for its applicability to aircraft design. It has since been applied successfully to an array of equipment and systems issues in the continuous process and batch-processing industries. When designing an aircraft, aerospace engineers naturally are very interested in learning the answer to this question, What *could* be the effects on the equipment and the entire aircraft if a component would fail? It is important to emphasize the term *could* because traditional FMEA focuses on what *might* go wrong, not what *has* gone wrong. Whenever one is dealing with probabilities, the analysis is also dealing with subjectivity. When one is forecasting, he or she is dealing with uncertainty. When dealing with uncertainty, one relies on the best data available to narrow the range of uncertainty.

From a statistical standpoint and scientific approach, FMEA can be defined as "a procedure by which each potential (anticipated) failure mode in a system is analyzed to determine the result or its effect on the system and to classify each potential failure mode according to severity" (Norbert S. Jagodzinski, personal communication, July 2003). With this definition in mind, one must break down the system (the aircraft) into its manageable subsystems. A typical aircraft would have many subsystems, but for this example think of just a few highly abbreviated ones, such as the wing assembly, instrumentation system, fuselage, engines, and so forth (Figure 4.1).

The analysis would look at each of these subsystems and determine what failure events might occur and, if failures did occur, what could be the effects (Latino and Latino, 2002). Look at the simple example from Table 4.1, the turbine engine subsystem. One begins by listing all the failure modes that might occur on the turbine engines. In this case, one might determine that a turbine blade could fracture. The next step is to ask what might be the effects on other items in the turbine engine subsystem. If the blade were to release, it could fracture the other turbine blades. The effects on the entire system, the aircraft as a whole, would be loss of the engine and reduced power and control of the aircraft. The process begins examining the severity of the failure mode, using a simple scale of 1 to 10, where 1 is the least severe and 10 is the most severe. This has been simplified for the present explanation, but a traditional FMEA analyst would have specific criteria defined for each level of severity from 1 through 10. In this example, assume that losing a turbine blade would constitute a severity of 8. Next one has to make a

TABLE 4.1. TRADITIONAL FMEA SAMPLE.

Subsystem	Mode	Effects on Other Items	Effects on Entire System	Severity	Probability	Criticality
Turbine engine	Cracked blade	If blade releases, it could fracture other blades	Loss of one engine, reduced power & control	8	.02	0.16

FIGURE 4.1. AIRCRAFT SUBSYSTEM DIAGRAM.

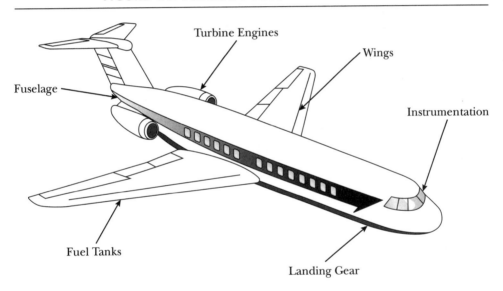

probability rating; this means collecting enough data to determine the relative probability of this occurrence, given the design of the aircraft. Assume for this example that the probability is .02, or 2 percent. The last step is to multiply the severity times the probability to get a criticality rating. In this case that rating would be calculated as follows:

$$8 \times .02 = 0.16$$
$$\text{Severity} \times \text{Probability} = \text{Criticality}$$

This sample criticality equation finds that this line item in the FMEA has a criticality rating of 0.16. This process would be repeated for all the failure modes in the turbine engines and all the other major subsystems. This seems like, and is, an immense amount of work. And for what? For passenger safety of course! A frequent flier truly appreciates the efforts these designers go to for passenger safety. For a typical aircraft it may take fifty to one hundred man-years to complete a traditional FMEA on a new aircraft design.

This brings up another key cultural difference between the application of FMEA in aerospace and in health care. Will it be culturally acceptable to allocate fifty to one hundred man-years to doing a traditional FMEA on a typical health care system? It is not acceptable in most industry as workforces are lean and budgets are tight. Doing such an analysis is not seen as revenue generating, therefore companies typically cannot apply such resources.

Applying Traditional FMEA to Health Care

The driving force behind the use of FMEA in health care is JCAHO. As is usually the case, most incentives to apply new technologies are imbedded in regulatory requirements or guidelines. Regulatory compliance is usually the motivator. This is a universal paradigm, not just one found in health care. One can ask, If the regulation or guideline did not exist (along with its penalties for noncompliance), would the technology be implemented? Currently, JCAHO FMEA guidelines (Standard LD.5.2) describe the following steps:

1. Select one high-risk process (most frequently occurring types of sentinel events and patient safety risk factors).
2. Conduct *failure modes analysis.*
3. Pinpoint undesirable variation with adverse effects on patients.
4. Carry out process redesign, testing, and implementation.
5. Measure effectiveness of change.

These guidelines express what is necessary to be in compliance. Knowing this, how does one apply FMEA to be compliant and also to get a quantum benefit in improved patient safety? Too often what is seen is a great amount of resources allocated to ensure compliance with regulatory statutes but no real benefit passed on to the organization. For example, in industry it is commonplace for various personnel to attend certain safety courses for a predefined number of hours per year. Compliance is that one spends a certain number of hours in a classroom. The problem with this is that the material is often stagnant; the person is seeing and hearing the same things he or she saw and heard last year. The person is still in compliance; however, the organization has not benefited. If anything, it has lost

TABLE 4.2. FMEA LINE ITEM SAMPLE.

Item	Failure Mode	Effect on Other Items	Effect on Entire System	Severity (S)	Probability (P)	Criticality (C = S × P)
Adverse events involving children	Wrong dose	Length of stay	Malpractice claims	7	3	21

because it is paying the student a day's wage to sit in a classroom so he or she can be deemed compliant.

So what would it take to be compliant under the JCAHO guidelines? Falling back on the aircraft FMEA example, look at a hypothetical case involving traditional FMEA on the following high-risk process: adverse events involving children. The failure modes and effects analysis (FMEA) spreadsheet might look like the example in Table 4.2. When one looks at the values applied to the severities and probabilities, one can see clearly the subjectivity noted earlier. Several standards exist for applying such values, so the user must choose which is acceptable for his or her application. For example, consider the following set of health care standards, established by the VA National Center for Patient Safety (Veterans Administration, 2002).

Sample Severity Classifications

- Catastrophic event (10)
  "A failure that may cause death or system loss"
- Major event (7)
  "A failure that may cause a high degree of customer dissatisfaction"
- Moderate event (4)
  "Failure that can be overcome with modifications to the process or product, but there is minor performance loss"
- Minor event (1)
  "Failure that will not be noticeable to the customer and would not affect delivery of the service or product"

Sample Probability Classifications

- Frequent (4)
  "Likely to occur immediately or within a short period (may happen several times in one year)"

FIGURE 4.2. TYPICAL FMEA HAZARD SCORING MATRIX.

	Severity			
	Catastrophic	Major	Moderate	Minor
Probability	16	12	8	4
	12	9	6	3
	8	6	4	2
	4	3	2	1

Source: Veterans Administration, 2002, fig. 5.

- Occasional (3)
   "Probably will occur (may happen several times in 1 to 2 years)"
- Uncommon (2)
   "Possible to occur (may happen sometime in 2 to 5 years)"
- Remote (1)
   "Unlikely to occur (may happen sometime in 5 to 30 years)"

The spreadsheet is full of modes that could occur and their subjective criticalities to the overall process. What can one do with it? This is where many different points of view come into play. To be in compliance with JCAHO guidelines, one must apply a rationale to determine which modes it would be most prudent to look at more closely in order to learn their causes. Again, many models are out there, and users must determine what is acceptable for their circumstances. Some use an FMEA *hazard scoring matrix,* such as the example in Figure 4.2.

Others prefer the approach of applying the Pareto principle, or the 80/20 rule as it is commonly referred to. This is where one can identify those modes that are accountable for most risk. Commonly, around 20 percent of the modes will be accountable for around 80 percent of the risk. The deliverable of this approach is the identification of the *significant few* (Latino and Latino, 2002, p. 46). The significant few chart may look something like Figure 4.3.

FMEA and Consequential Thinking

Given the origin and intent of FMEA, what benefits can one seek and what pitfalls should one avoid when applying it in health care? The response to this question involves *consequential thinking.* Understanding the intent and environment for which the original FMEA was created and also understanding where one intends

FIGURE 4.3. SIGNIFICANT FEW CHART.

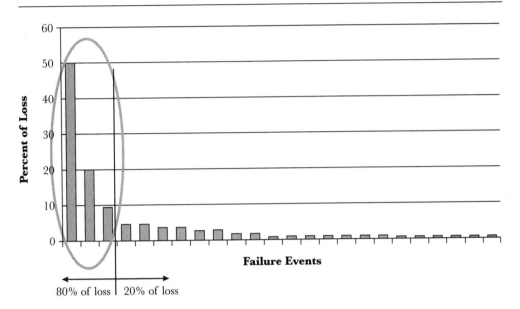

to apply it in health care, what other considerations should be taken into account?

- The taxonomy of terms
- The scope of the analysis
- The quantification of outcomes
- The leveraging of peer review protections

Considering the items in this list brings out some of the key cultural differences between a manufacturing operation and a health care environment. It is useful to look at each of these items in further detail.

Taxonomy of Terms

In today's litigious society, liability is of the utmost concern—especially in health care. One must always be concerned about how various types of information might be construed in the different contexts. Consider the connotations of the following terms:

FTA: *fault* tree analysis or *failure* tree analysis

FMEA: *failure* modes and effects analysis

FMECA: *failure* modes, effects, and *criticality* analysis

RCFA: root cause *failure* analysis

One can plainly see the commonalities among these terms. One can also see the potentially offensive nature of these terms when used in health care. Granted, these terms are acceptable in an engineering environment. After all, engineers at times are troubleshooters, determining why equipment and processes fail. The term *failure* is often associated with mechanical failure, or equipment-related failure. However, in health care a failure may involve an action that results in death. No one would like to be associated with a failure in a health care culture. A failure in a manufacturing plant may involve the loss of substantial money, but in health care it may involve loss of life. For these reasons, when applying these FMEA concepts to health care, one should consider changing potentially offensive terms to more acceptable terms. For instance:

> *FTA* may be changed to *logic tree analysis.*
>
> *FMEA* and *FMECA* may be changed to *opportunity analysis.*
>
> *RCFA* may be changed to *root cause analysis.*

The outcomes of these processes should not change because the methodology has not changed, only the names are different. What should also be different is the acceptance of the method based on its name and the legal protection that the name provides.

Scope of the Analysis

Under the current JCAHO guidelines, an FMEA is required to be conducted on one (1) high-risk process (most frequently occurring types of sentinel events and patient safety risk factors). Who determines which process is the highest risk one? Certainly a conflict may develop in this area, with quality, risk, and claims management functions differing on which process has the highest risk or priority. Even within a single discipline such as risk management, how does one decide which has the highest risk? Should one restrict FMEAs to sentinel events? Should adverse drug events (ADEs) or near misses be included in this category? One can see the dilemma. Also, from the legal standpoint, if one restricts FMEA to sentinel events as the high-risk process, does this raise a risk of vulnerability to litigation? If an ADE occurs that did not come up in the FMEA on the sentinel events, could the healthcare organization be liable because it should have looked at that process? What if one overlooked an event that should have been included in an FMEA, what are the consequences? Although this may seem cumbersome, there are costs associated with noncompliance and the potential for claims activity as a consequence of omitting events or items in an FMEA. After completing an

FMEA and determining the significant few, which process should be examined with root cause analysis (RCA)? If one selects the wrong one to examine first, and an incident occurs in one of the processes that was not selected, what are the consequences?

Suggested here is a path of thought that forces one to consider consequential thinking. What will be the potential consequences of such action, and is the response appropriate under the scenarios considered?

The quality, risk, and claims management functions all have a unique focus and purpose within a health care environment. With these unique perspectives come different priorities. A traditional FMEA conducted on a process in the risk management area and one done on a process in the claims management area will certainly yield diametrically different outcomes. Risk management explores what could happen and claims management is interested in learning from what has happened. Knowing this difference in perspective, it is imperative to provide a justifiable rationale for what was included or excluded in the scope of the analysis.

An array of definitions is used in these analyses. For example:

- Any event or condition that results in a sentinel event (risk management perspective)
- Any event or condition that results in an adverse drug event (risk management perspective)
- Any event or condition that results in a near miss (quality management perspective)
- Any event or condition that results in an extended length of stay (claims perspective)
- Any event or condition that results in a medication order process error (claims perspective)

Quantification of Outcomes

Traditional FMEA measures the criticality of certain events to the process (probability × severity = criticality). As discussed earlier, the term *criticality* itself could pose a problem. A better term to use may be *rank prioritization number* (RPN). This is less offensive and less threatening and accomplishes the same thing.

What about those times when one uses FMEA retrospectively? That is, the FMEA would be modified and applied to historical events. Under these conditions one could use a variation of the FMEA concept and apply it to fields such as quality, risk, and claims management. The variation used for this purpose in this chapter is called LEAP™ Opportunity Analysis (Reliability Center, 2002).

FIGURE 4.4. LEAP NEW ANALYSIS WIZARD.

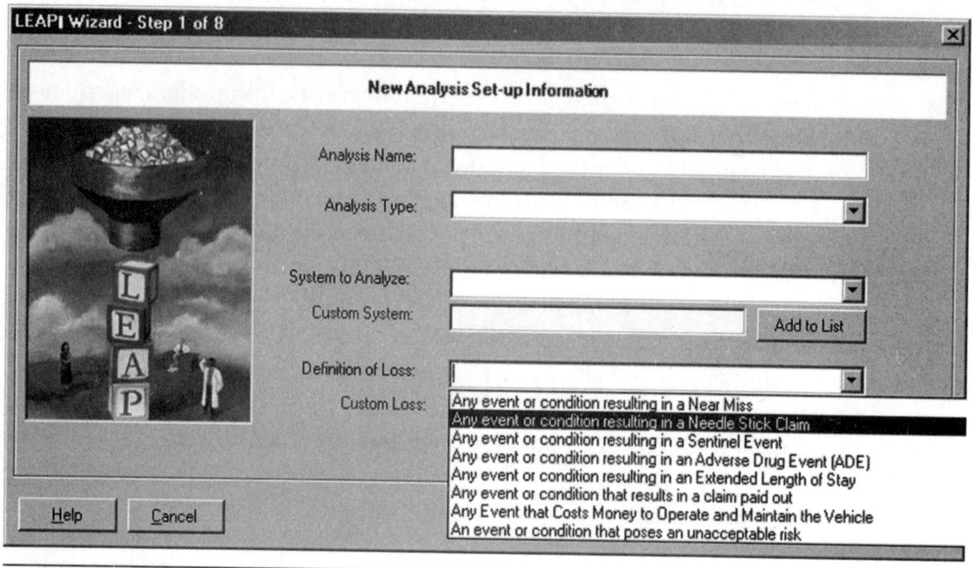

LEAP Wizard - Step 1 of 8   ☒

New Analysis Set-up Information

Analysis Name:

Analysis Type:

System to Analyze:

Custom System: Add to List

Definition of Loss:

Custom Loss: Any event or condition resulting in a Near Miss
                Any event or condition resulting in a Needle Stick Claim
                Any event or condition resulting in a Sentinel Event
                Any event or condition resulting in an Adverse Drug Event (ADE)
                Any event or condition resulting in an Extended Length of Stay
                Any event or condition that results in a claim paid out
                Any Event that Costs Money to Operate and Maintain the Vehicle
                An event or condition that poses an unacceptable risk

Help   Cancel

Source: Reliability Center, 2002.

Recognizing that there are other approaches for this purpose, this methodology uses either probabilistic or historical data in the analyses. "New Analysis Wizard" (Figure 4.4) allows users to configure the analysis setup to their specifications.

The uniqueness here is that the users determine whether they wish to conduct a traditional FMEA with probabilistic data to meet regulatory requirements or whether they wish to use the system for identifying opportunities that are outside the scope of simply complying with regulatory requirements. The latter use is referred to as *opportunity analysis,* and it employs historical data to sift out past trends that represent future opportunities (Figure 4.5).

What is so special about using historical data rather than strictly probabilistic data? With historical data, one is basing projections on factual information, not suspect data. For instance, one may want to focus the analysis on all claims paid out over the past two-year period. Such data likely reside somewhere in current information systems, although they may be scattered among various systems. Once one knows the scope of the analysis (claims systems) and the definition of loss (claims paid), one can determine how one wants the loss measured. In this instance, one may choose to use dollars or one could use severity of impact (Figure 4.6). The point is that the selection is based on the nature of analysis and the circumstances that surround it.

FIGURE 4.5. NEW ANALYSIS WIZARD (STEP 3).

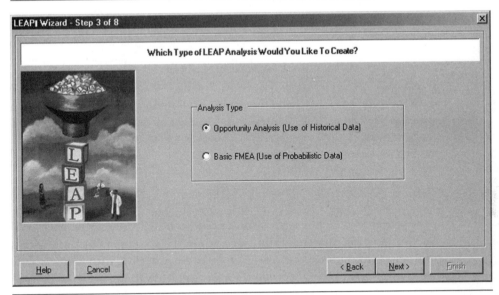

Source: Reliability Center, 2002.

FIGURE 4.6. NEW ANALYSIS WIZARD (STEP 4).

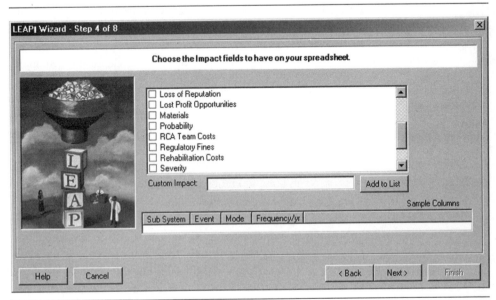

Source: Reliability Center, 2002.

When a potential liability is involved, one may choose to use severity of impact. For example, a weighted scale may be applied where

> 1 = Claim paid was substantial.
> 2 = Claim paid was moderate.
> 3 = Claim paid was minor.

Remember, the key here is that the *analyst* is configuring the focus of the analysis. In this scenario one could also choose to use actual dollars paid out. The focus is at the discretion of the analyst.

The reason for selecting one method of measuring outcomes over another is very important because it becomes the business rationale for why one chooses to focus in one area rather than another. Think about how losses can be measured. One can measure their severity through a weighted scale. One can measure dollars associated with each event, such as attorney's fees, RCA team costs, labor costs, material costs, lost profit opportunity costs, loss of reputation costs, rebranding costs, and many, many other costs. One should give this part of the analysis extensive thought so that the analysis serves its intended purposes.

Although this process is being referred to as *opportunity analysis* (in order, as explained earlier, to use a term that emphasizes process benefits), it is nothing more than modified FMEA.

To continue using the LEAP approach after setting up the new analysis, the next step is to map out the process flow using a process flowchart. Assume one is looking at a blood bank center. The scope of the analysis is that center and the definition of loss is *severity of injury.* How can one measure losses? One develops a weighted severity scale ranging from 1 to 10, with 10 being the most severe injury. One would be interested in knowing the extended length of stay for each injury, measured in days. The next step is to take the sum of these impacts, or losses, and multiply the result by the frequency of occurrence (extrapolated over a year's time). Working under these conditions, one looks for data needed in the process and includes the information in the LEAP Opportunity Analysis format. The process flowchart might look like the one in Figure 4.7. A LEAP Opportunity Analysis worksheet might look like the one in Figure 4.8.

What should one do with the data collected and put into this format? Which events should be the subject of a root cause analysis (RCA)? LEAP uses a variation of the Pareto principle, the 80/20 rule. When one selects the "calculate significant few button" (Figure 4.8), the program identifies the events that account for 80 percent or more of the total losses identified (Figure 4.9). The business case or justification for doing RCA on these specific events is related to identified (factual) impacts on the organization. Continuing with the example of the blood bank, the

FIGURE 4.7. PROCESS FLOW DIAGRAM.

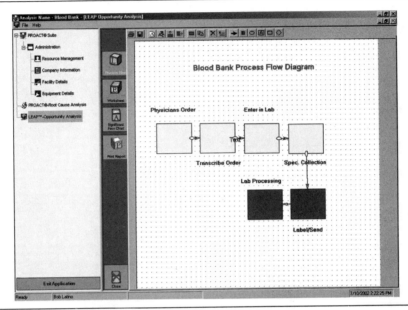

Source: Reliability Center, 2002.

FIGURE 4.8. OPPORTUNITY ANALYSIS WORKSHEET.

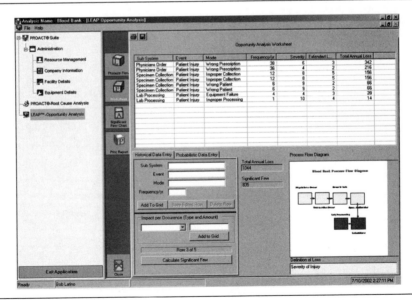

Source: Reliability Center, 2002.

FIGURE 4.9. SIGNIFICANT FEW EVENTS.

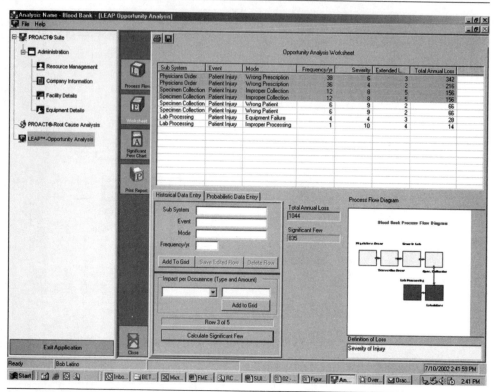

Source: Reliability Center, 2002.

significant few items may be graphically represented as shown in Figure 4.10. This is the type and form of information that one would report to management. It possesses all the characteristics needed to make it acceptable: regulatory compliance, a factual basis, a focused and disciplined approach, and a justification tied to what is important to the organization. The last step is to use a function in the software that enables the user to print the full report. (Figure 4.11).

Variations of the traditional FMEA can thus be used to benefit all disciplines in an organization. The next step is to leverage peer review.

Leveraging Peer Review Protections

Earlier the importance of terminology when trying to implement new technologies in the health care environment was discussed. The question for health care is, in today's litigious environment, is there a "tolerance" for new terms?

FIGURE 4.10. SIGNIFICANT FEW CHART.

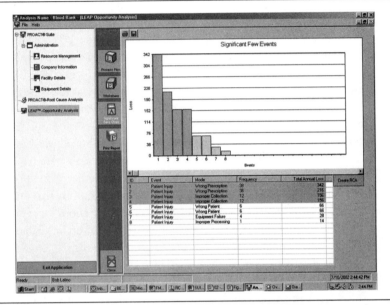

Source: Reliability Center, 2002.

FIGURE 4.11. LEAP REPORT.

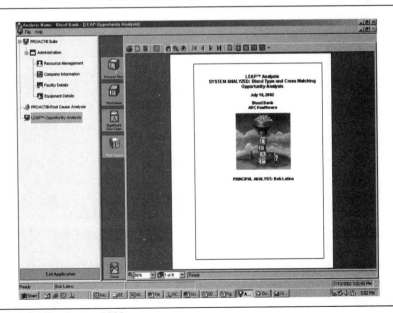

Source: Reliability Center, 2002.

(Rozovsky, 2002). The health care field is continually faced with public pressure for increased patient safety and with federal, state, and local regulations that support public opinion in this area. It is this mix that forces the health care field to be acutely aware of legal responsibilities at all times. What if one's FMEA chart and background information were subject to discovery and admissibility? What if one uses FMEA as provided in the JCAHO guidelines and only works on the highest priority identified? What if an event occurs that was identified in a past FMEA, and the health care organization had taken no proactive corrective actions because its priority was low in the analysis? These are serious questions in the health care environment where results of actions may be scrutinized from a legal standpoint. Even the terminology issue discussed earlier, which may seem trivial at first glance, might lead to a plaintiff's counsel saying something like this: "You see, ladies and gentlemen of the jury, they knew that the potential for this event could occur because it was identified in their FMEA. Then they chose to do nothing about it!" True or not, that may be the spin that would be put on an earlier action.

To this end, techniques such as FMEA, FTA, FMECA, and even opportunity analysis should be used as part of an overall strategy to maximally leverage peer review protection. Structured and disciplined approaches like these are very useful to peer reviews. When such disciplined investigative techniques are used, they will require the regimented acquisition of data to support hypotheses and ultimately conclusions. Under peer review protections, these data will not be discoverable, so there will be an incentive to be credible and thorough. Peer review protections should encourage such analyses to be open, no matter what the findings, in the interest of overall patient safety. Without such protections, data collection tends to be limited, and what is collected may be diluted with watered-down wording to protect individuals and the organization from litigation.

In a broader context, when writing up reports for FMEA and RCA, less offensive terminology should be used that is oriented toward quality improvement. Such actions will make the report more acceptable within the organization as well as within the legal world.

It should also be noted that projected risks are the focal point when conducting FMEAs. There is no need to apply quantitative dollar values to such situations. Attaching dollar values to risk events in a report may lead to real or perceived catastrophic decision errors. People may say or find that the organization chose to implement corrective actions for the events likely to be most costly to the organization rather than the ones that posed the most risk to the patients. Using consequential thinking tools, one can foresee and avoid the occasion for this objection.

The intent in this chapter has been to show that failure modes and effects analysis can be used in virtually any situation to the advantage of the organization. It does not have to be applied only in accordance with JCAHO guidelines.

An organization could do an opportunity analysis on any process that has resulted in, for example:

- Needle stick claims
- Blood redraws in the ER
- Claims paid out in general
- Customer dissatisfaction
- Near misses

These are events that have occurred. They are factual findings. Applying values to these events may be more acceptable *because* these selections have already occurred. Anyone could research the details and determine the costs associated with these events each time one occurs. That is, from a discoverability standpoint, the information is out there already. Through FMEA or RCA the information is organized in a manner that permits health care organizations to learn the most prudent areas in which to allocate lean resources.

Peer review protections are in place because organizations need honest and accurate information in order to understand the root causes of undesirable events. All undesirable events have some roots embedded in flawed human decision-making processes. Unfortunately, many organizational cultures still find satisfaction in the witch-hunting philosophy, the theory that it is useful to make an example of someone or some group for making an improper decision. What the advocates of witch hunting may not realize is that true root cause analysis involves understanding *why* people make the decisions that they do. Certainly, the great preponderance of health care providers do not intend to make mistakes that will result in a patient safety issue. In order to stop undesirable outcomes, it is important to understand the logic mechanisms that led to a string of errors. The fact is that the organization is responsible for implementing the management systems that encourage better decision making by its personnel. Systems that establish and maintain policies, procedures, practices, guidelines, training approaches, purchasing habits, and the like are designed to help managers, leaders and workers make better decisions in work environments. These are the *laws* of the organization. One may ask, however, with technology advancing at a staggering rate, are organizations able to keep up with the support systems that should ensure the success of new approaches?

An example reinforces this point. Many people remember what happened when their facility installed new computer systems or software or diagnostic equipment. Some did not receive training on the proper use of the equipment. Procedures were not updated to include information about the new equipment or software. The result may have been that a "cost-saving measure" ended up costing more than the original amount to be saved. For example, assume that a pharmacy gave the wrong version of an antibiotic to a patient who then had a serious allergic reaction to the drug. This resulted in a claim. The reason that the pharmacy dispensed this particular medication was most interesting. The pharmacy had been instructed by the organization's finance department to reduce costs by 10 percent, as part of a continuous improvement effort. As a result the formulary was curbed to include fewer versions of a particular antibiotic family. In the long run, the pharmacy cost the organization a substantial amount of money.

Conclusion

Failure modes and effects analysis offers health care organizations the opportunity to better understand risk. To be successful one must consider several steps:

1. Seek to adopt a less offensive taxonomy of terms when delving into the world of understanding why things go wrong.
2. Treat analysis processes as quality improvement processes.
3. Educate in-house users in the FMEA methodology, not just in a software package; develop their unbiased analytical skills.
4. Emphasize strict adherence to the discipline of the method and to maintaining the associated documentation to prove the results.
5. Leverage peer review protections to the maximum.
6. Train legal counsel so that they better understand the analytical process being used and how it generates its findings. This will prepare them to better protect the organization (while letting it do its job with excellence).
7. Measure numbers at the end of the process, not at the front.
8. Always practice consequential thinking. Using FMEA, opportunity analysis, and especially RCA will sharpen this skill over time.
9. Use the LEAP Opportunity Analysis or a similar approach to explore various applications to improve the systems within the organization.
10. Recognize that witch hunting is *not* a form of scientific analysis (much to the dismay of popular belief).

Even though many issues discussed here appear complex, it is the role of those who must put patient safety compliance into practice to break paradigms of complexity into manageable components. Analysts must seek to identify the true opportunities that exist in a fashion that protects the patient in the end and protects the organization's ability to stay in business and provide safe services to the community that everyone in the organization knows and enjoys.

References

Latino, R. J., and Latino, K. C. *Root Cause Analysis: Improving Performance for Bottom-Line Results.* Boca Raton: CRC Press, 2002.

Reliability Center. LEAP™. A module in the PROACT Suite. Hopewell, Va.: Reliability Center, 2002.

Rozovsky, F. A. Presentation to the Virginia Chapter of the American Society for Healthcare Risk Management (VASHRM), Williamsburg, Va., Feb. 2002.

Veterans Administration, National Center for Patient Safety. *Healthcare Failure Mode and Effect Analysis Course Materials (HFMEA™).* [http://www.patientsafety.gov/HFMEA.html]. 2002.

CHAPTER FIVE

MEDICATION ERROR REDUCTION

Voluntary and Regulatory Oversight

David M. Benjamin
John P. Santell

"**M**odern health care presents the most complex safety challenge of any activity on earth. However, we have failed to design our systems for safety, relying instead on requiring individual error-free performance enforced by punishment, a strategy abandoned long ago by safer industries such as aviation and nuclear power." So say Lucian Leape and colleagues in a JAMA editorial (Leape and others, 1998). Indeed, when you stop to think about it, why is it that the connector fitting on the intravenous (IV) lines and the nasogastric (NG) tubes fit one another? And aren't you glad that anesthesia machines can no longer deliver an anesthetic gas unless the oxygen is running?

Unfortunately, when it comes to health care, Murphy's Law not only applies but leads one to the inescapable conclusion of Murphy's disciple, O'Brien, who said of his mentor, "Murphy is an optimist!" The problem is that Leape is right; modern health care is so complex that physicians, nurses, and pharmacists can no longer carry around in their heads all the information they need to practice their professions. Moreover, the health care system is designed not to prevent error but rather in a manner that places the responsibility of error prevention squarely on health care practitioners. There are still many common practices that can lead to unintended tragedy, such as allowing nurses access to harmful floor stock items like vials of concentrated potassium chloride (KCl), rather than restricting such items to the pharmacy or operating room pharmacy satellites. Concentrated potassium chloride is one of the three drugs used in lethal injection, and it definitely will adversely affect a patient in one's institution if it is given without proper dilution (see 2004 Patient Safety Goal 3a of the Joint Commission on Accreditation of Healthcare Organizations [JCAHO] in Exhibit 5.1). And there are other problem-prone practices. Many hospital pharmacies stock medications alphabetically, with the result that different products with similar-looking names (for example, Lamisil and Lamictal) are right next to each other on the shelf, leading at times to the dispensing of the wrong drug. According to data collected by the two medication error reporting programs of the United States Pharmacopeia (USP), confusion because of the similarity of drug names when either written or spoken (look-alike or sound-alike) accounts for approximately 5 to 15 percent of all reported errors (Hicks, Cousins, and Williams, 2003; USP, 2001). Still not convinced? Remember when omeprazole first came out on the market for the treatment of gastric hyperacidity? Its brand name then was Losec. After numerous prescriptions for Lasix 50 mg were mistakenly and unfortunately dispensed as Losec 50 mg, the manufacturer changed the brand name of the drug to Prilosec. This case signals a new awareness by manufacturers that product naming and labeling play a role in medication errors. Medical and medication errors are emerging from their cloak of invisibility, and health care is entering the age of self-critical analysis slowly. Organizations in the private sector like the National Patient Safety Foundation, the Institute for Healthcare Improvement, and the Leapfrog Group have joined governmental agencies like the Agency for Healthcare Research and Quality (AHRQ) and the Food and Drug Administration (FDA) in jumping on the ambulance en route to treating our ailing health care system.

What is the result of putting the practice of medicine under the microscope? Physicians, patient safety experts, systems engineers, and software manufacturers have identified many of the most common system errors and unsafe practices that occur in the health care setting and are in the process of redesigning systems to decrease the likelihood of making an error. In addition, our legislators have proposed new law, in the form of the Patient Safety and Quality Improvement Act, that not only encourages the reporting of medical and medication errors to newly designated *patient safety organizations* (PSOs) but also provides legal privilege for such documented reporting. According to this proposed Act, in order to be certified as a PSO an organization must meet certain specified criteria. It must conduct activities that improve patient safety and the quality of health care delivery. It must not have any conflicts of interest with its providers. The PSO must have appropriately trained staff, including licensed or certified medical professionals. The PSO cannot be a component of an insurance company. It must operate independently, and it must collect patient safety data in a standardized manner that permits valid comparisons of similar cases among similar providers.

EXHIBIT 5.1.   2004 JCAHO NATIONAL PATIENT SAFETY GOALS.

1. Improve the accuracy of patient identification.

   a. Use at least two patient identifiers (neither to be the patient's room number) whenever taking blood samples or administering medications or blood products.
   b. Prior to the start of any surgical or invasive procedure, conduct a final verification process, such as a "time out," to confirm the correct patient, procedure and site, using active—not passive—communication techniques.

2. Improve the effectiveness of communication among caregivers.

   a. Implement a process for taking verbal or telephone orders or critical test results that require a verification "read-back" of the complete order or test result by the person receiving the order or test result.
   b. Standardize the abbreviations, acronyms and symbols used throughout the organization, including a list of abbreviations, acronyms and symbols *not* to use.

3. Improve the safety of using high-alert medications.

   a. Remove concentrated electrolytes (including, but not limited to, potassium chloride, potassium phosphate, sodium chloride >0.9%) from patient care units.
   b. Standardize and limit the number of drug concentrations available in the organization.

4. Eliminate wrong-site, wrong-patient, wrong-procedure surgery.

   a. Create and use a preoperative verification process, such as a checklist, to confirm that appropriate documents (e.g., medical records, imaging studies) are available.
   b. Implement a process to mark the surgical site and involve the patient in the marking process.

5. Improve the safety of using infusion pumps.

   a. Ensure free-flow protection on all general-use and PCA (patient controlled analgesia) intravenous infusion pumps used in the organization.

6. Improve the effectiveness of clinical alarm systems.

   a. Implement regular preventive maintenance and testing of alarm systems.
   b. Assure that alarms are activated with appropriate settings and are sufficiently audible with respect to distances and competing noise within the unit.

7. Reduce the risk of health care–acquired infections.

   a. Comply with current CDC hand hygiene guidelines.
   b. Manage as sentinel events all identified cases of unanticipated death or major permanent loss of function associated with a health care–acquired infection.

Source: JCAHO, 2004.

It is to be hoped that in the near future, practitioners and hospitals no longer will need to be concerned that quality improvement investigations or root cause analyses will be used against them as evidence of negligence in any subsequent legal proceeding. Moreover, PSOs will have opportunities to analyze error reports and issue educational updates on the frequency and severity of reported medication errors. Programs currently in place already provide hospitals a way to measure (or compare) their improvement in medication safety and to determine where they have progressed and where more effort is still needed. Such programs will be of greatest value only if and when legislative protection for submitted data is enacted.

One such existing program is the U.S. Pharmacopeia's MEDMARX error reporting program, which facilitates analysis of medication errors in the institutional setting. This anonymous, confidential, deidentified, Internet-accessible program allows hospitals and other health care facilities to report, track, and share medication error data in a standardized format. MEDMARX uses the nationally recognized National Coordinating Council for Medication Error Reporting and Prevention (NCC MERP) taxonomy, which includes an index for categorizing error events by severity and outcome and allows the capture of both potential and *near-miss* events as well as harmful errors. This system for categorizing medication errors is summarized in Exhibit 5.2.

Recently, USP summarized data findings for the three-year period covering January 1, 1999, to December 31, 2001, (Santell, Hicks, McMeekin, and Cousins, 2003). During that period, USP examined 154,816 medication error records that were reported to the MEDMARX database. Errors labeled as Category C made up approximately 47 percent (72,000 out of 154,816) of the total. Category B was the next most frequently cited error category (32 percent). Records citing Category E errors occurred only 2.2 percent of the time. Category F errors occurred only 0.4 percent of the time (4 times per 1,000 errors). The most serious medication errors, in categories G, H, and I, occurred only 1, 3, and 1 time(s) in 10,000, respectively, and medication errors in categories E through I, representing all harmful errors and those requiring intervention or hospitalization, occurred 2.63 percent of the time overall.

Unfortunately, many hospitals have medication safety reporting systems (whether for medication errors or adverse drug reactions) that suffer from inadequate or inconsistent data capture. This results in great underreporting and causes frustration for those charged with analyzing and communicating the findings because key data elements often are missing. Other hospitals are diligent about collecting complete data but are uncertain how best to use those data. To help transform data into useful information, USP has constructed a medication safety initiative model for hospitals (Figure 5.1). The model is based on USP's work with

EXHIBIT 5.2.   NCC MERP ERROR CATEGORY INDEX FOR SEVERITY LEVELS AND OUTCOMES.

No error

- Category A: Circumstances or events that have the capacity to cause error.

Error, no harm

- Category B: An error occurred, but the error did not reach the patient.
- Category C: An error occurred that reached the patient but did not cause patient harm.
- Category D: An error occurred that reached the patient and required monitoring to confirm that it resulted in no harm to the patient or required intervention to preclude harm.

Error, harm

- Category E: An error occurred that may have contributed to or resulted in temporary harm to the patient and required intervention.
- Category F: An error occurred that may have contributed to or resulted in temporary harm to the patient and required initial or prolonged hospitalization.
- Category G: An error occurred that may have contributed to or resulted in permanent patient harm.
- Category H: An error occurred that required an intervention necessary to sustain life.

Error, death

- Category I: An error occurred that may have contributed to or resulted in patient's death.

Source: National Coordinating Council for Medication Error Reporting and Prevention, 2001.

practitioners and health systems, work with error reporting programs, and experience with the issues of medication safety. It consists of four stages that deal with the environment and culture, data collection, data analysis, and assessment of the impact of actions taken in response to errors.

Published data from national error reporting programs such as MEDMARX, accompanied by safety models and technology, are becoming more available as risk management tools to improve the safety of health care. CEOs often seek a business case for patient safety and for supportive tools like MEDMARX. But the real question they should ask is how can one afford not to have some of these new advances in quality improvement and risk assessment? The next step is to get the word out to every practitioner and hospital administrator that patient safety tools are available and need only be implemented in their health care facilities and medical offices in order to work.

FIGURE 5.1. USP MEDICATION SAFETY INITIATIVE MODEL.

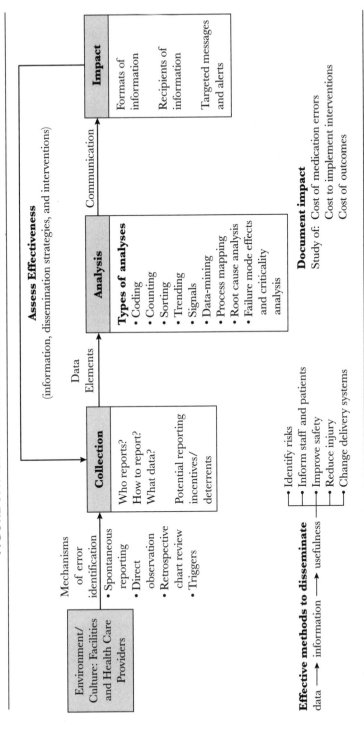

Source: USP, 2002a.

What about cost? How can one afford electronic medical records or computerized prescriber order entry (CPOE) or clinical pharmacists on every floor to assist physicians with drug therapy decisions and nurses with medication-related questions? Leape and others (1997) reported that the use of clinical pharmacists to assist physicians in selecting and prescribing medications reduced adverse drug reactions by 66 percent and was reported to have the potential to save one intensive care unit an estimated $270,000 over the course of a year, based on an estimated saving of $4,685 per preventable adverse drug event. In 1998, Bates and others demonstrated that CPOE could decrease adverse drug experiences (ADEs) by 84 percent and serious medication errors by 55 percent. Decreasing medication errors saves money for the hospital and the health care system in general, to say nothing about avoiding the costs of litigation.

Medication Error Reduction in the Institutional Setting

In the institutional setting the *medication use process* (MUP) begins with writing the medication order and ends with monitoring the effects of the prescribed drug on the patient. The process can be schematized as illustrated in Figure 5.2. This schematic makes it apparent that getting the right drug to the right patient requires excellent communication skills (both oral and written) among the members of the health care team. Unfortunately, language is inherently inexact, and communication errors form the basis for many medication errors and therapeutic misadventures (Benjamin, 2001b; USP, 2002b).

The danger of poorly written communication has been illustrated in several, well-publicized cases. For example, when *Boston Globe* health reporter Betsy Lehman received a fatal, fourfold overdose of her cyclophosphamide chemotherapy, it opened everyone's eyes to the dangers inherent in prescription writing. The order had been written as, "4 g/sq m over four days" (that is, four grams per square meter over 4 days). The intention was that one-quarter of the dose (1 g/sq m) be given once daily for four days, but the order was misinterpreted, and 4 g/sq m

FIGURE 5.2. SCHEMATIC OF MEDICATION USE PROCESS IN THE INSTITUTIONAL SETTING.

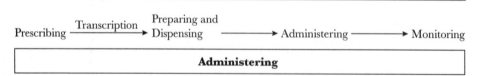

were given as a single lethal dose (ECRI, 2000). Complete, accurate, and appropriately communicated medication orders are essential in reducing medication errors. One of JCAHO's National Patient Safety Goals (Exhibit 5.1, Goal 2) advocates written policies aimed at minimizing errors in the communication of medication orders, specifically in the areas of verbal (or telephone) orders and the use of abbreviations. The goal recommends developing a standardized list of abbreviations, including abbreviations that should *not* be used because they can be confusing (see, for example, Table 5.1).

In 2002, data from USP's MEDMARX program (Hicks, Cousins, and Williams, 2003) tracked error reports, listing seven different communication-related causes of error: (1) communication, (2) verbal order, (3) brand names sound alike, (4) brand and generic names sound alike, (5) generic names sound alike, (6) abbreviations, and (7) nonmetric units used. Over 13 percent (26,386 out of 192,477) of all reported errors were associated with these *communication selections*, with the majority of the errors (nearly 63 percent) reaching the patient. Communication selections were reported in 7 out of every 20 reported fatal errors (35 percent) during 2002.

The way health care professionals communicate drug information varies considerably from hospital to hospital, floor to floor, and unit to unit. Patterns of communication in health care are primarily *conversational* (casual) rather than *computational* (analytical) (Coiera, 2000)—a style that in some situations undermines patient safety. Additional confounding factors, such as organizational processes, policies, and procedures, further contribute to the extent and scope of the problem. In the institutional setting the process of getting the medication "from the pen to the patient" may involve more than twenty individual steps, in contrast to the simplicity of prescribing for a patient in the outpatient setting, where the prescriber either calls, faxes, scans, or e-mails the prescription directly to the pharmacy or gives the prescription directly to the patient for presentation at the pharmacy. If there are twenty steps involved in getting the medicine to the patient, then there are twenty opportunities to make an error. Simplifying the system immediately helps. Even reducing the number of steps from twenty to nineteen reduces the possibility of making an error by 5 percent. Moreover, health care today is truly a team effort. No single health care professional can carry out all the steps by himself or herself. Physicians, nurses, and pharmacists must rely on each other as well as on specially trained clerks, nursing assistants, pharmacy technicians, and other hospital employees to perform their duties.

The complexity of the MUP in hospitals may be the reason why studies funded by the AHRQ revealed that 39 to 49 percent of medication errors at large hospitals occurred at the physician-prescribing stage of the process. Nursing

TABLE 5.1. POTENTIALLY DANGEROUS ABBREVIATIONS.

Abbreviation	Intended Meaning	Potential Misinterpretation	Recommendations
.5	One-half	May be read as 5	Use leading zero and write "0.5"
>	Greater than	May be confused with < (lesser than)	Write out the meaning
<	Less than	May be confused with > (greater than)	Write out the meaning
μg	Micrograms	May be interpreted as mg (milligrams)	Write "mcg"
¼ NS	Quarter-strength saline	May be interpreted as 0.45% saline	Write "0.225% sodium chloride"
½ NS	Half-strength saline	May be interpreted as 0.225% saline	Write "0.45% sodium chloride"
½ mg	0.5 mg	1.5 mg may be given to patient	Spell out "one-half" or use decimal ("0.5 mg")
1 Amp	One ampoule	1 milligram; may confuse size with strength	Write exact dose
12.0	Twelve	May be read as 120	Don't use trailing zero; write "12"
2–4 mg	2 mg up to 4 mg of medication to be given	May be read as 24 mg	Don't use hyphen; write "2 mg to 4 mg"
3lbs	3 pounds	May be read as 31 pounds	Spell out "pounds"
40 of K (verbal order)	40 mEq KCl (potassium chloride)	May be interpreted as Vitamin K 40 mg	Convey full name of product
5 ASA	5-acetylsalicylic acid (Mesalamine) suppository	May be interpreted as aspirin suppository, 5 grains	Write out generic name
AU AS AD	Both ears Left ear Right ear	Confused with optic route for administration	Write out "both ears" Write out "left ear" Write out "right ear"
CC or Cc	Cubic centimeter	May be mistaken for "U" (units) when poorly written	Use metric system "mL" or write out "milliliters"
CHG in saline	Chlorhexidine gluconate in saline		Write out generic name
D/C or DC	Discharge or discontinue	May be misinterpreted	Write out "discharge" or "discontinue"
D/C PT or DC PT	Discontinue physical therapy or discharge patient	May be misinterpreted	Write out intended meaning

TABLE 5.1. (*CONTINUED*)

Abbreviation	Intended Meaning	Potential Misinterpretation	Recommendations
DTaP	Vaccine for diphtheria, tetanus, acellular pertussis	May be confused with DTP	
FUDR	Fludarabine	May be interpreted as floxuridine	Write out complete drug product name—generic or trade
GM-CSF	Leukine	May be entered as G-CSF (Neupogen)	Write out complete product name—generic or trade
H	Humalog	May be interpreted as Humulin R	Write out complete product name
HC oint	Hydrocortisone ointment		
HCTZ	Hydrochlorothiazide	May be confused with hydrocortisone	Write out complete product name—generic or trade
HIB	Haemophilus influenzae B	May be confused with hepatitis B (HEP-B)	Write out generic name
HIB	Haemophilus influenzae B	May be confused with hepatitis B immune globulin (H-Big)	
PTN	Phenytoin	May be interpreted with multiple meanings	Write out generic name
IV	Intravenous or (4)	May be misinterpreted	Write out intended meaning
Hs or hs	Every night or half-strength	May be interpreted with multiple meanings; may be interpreted as every hour	Write out "every night" or "half strength"
Humalog, 2 unit qac	Humalog, 2 units, before each meal	Humalog, 2 units, every morning (q.am)	Write out completely
i/d	Once daily	May be read as TID	Write out "once daily"
L insulin	Lente insulin or Lantus insulin	May be misinterpreted	Write out generic or trade name
$MgSO_4$ or $MgSO_4$	Magnesium sulfate	May be confused with morphine sulfate	Write out complete product name—generic or trade
MMC	Mutamycin	Unapproved abbreviation	Write out complete product name—generic or trade
MS03	Morphine sulfate	May be confused with magnesium sulfate	Write out full name

(Continued)

TABLE 5.1.   POTENTIALLY DANGEROUS ABBREVIATIONS. (*CONTINUED*)

Abbreviation	Intended Meaning	Potential Misinterpretation	Recommendations
NO	Nitroglycerin ointment	May be read as mo	Write out generic name
OD	Right eye	May be interpreted as once daily	Write out "right eye" or "once daily"
OJ	Orange juice	May be interpreted as OD or OS	Write out "orange juice"
Oxy-IR		IR may be interpreted as 1–2	Write out generic name
per os	Oral route of administration	May be read as per OS (left eye)	Write "orally" or "by mouth" or "P.O."
PH	Pharmacy to dose	May be confused with PTT	Write out complete instructions; do not abbreviate
Pm or PM	Night dose	May be confused with prn	Write "nightly"
PMV	Passiy Muir Value	May be confused with prenatal vitamins	Write out intended meaning
PPN	Peripheral parenteral nutrition	May be interpreted as TPN (total parenteral nutrition)	Write out intended meaning
QD or qd	Every day	May be read as qid	Write out "daily"
QOD or qod	Every other day	May be confused with qid (four times daily)	Write out "every other day"
Q6	Every 6 hours	May be confused with qD (every day)	Write "hours" after entry
QD-HS	Daily at hour of sleep	May be confused as QD & HS	Avoid hyphens and write out
QDx2	Every day for 2 days	May be confused with bid (twice daily)	Write "daily for 2 days only"
QID or qid	4 times daily	May be confused with once daily	Spell out frequency
Sq or sc	Subcutaneous	The "q" may be read as meaning "every"	Write "subq"
SS or Ss	Sliding scale	May be confused with one-half	Write out "sliding scale"
TAC	Tetracaine, adrenaline, cocaine	May be confused with triamcinolone	Write out generic name
TAC	Triamcinolone	May be confused with Tetracaine, adrenaline, cocaine	Write out generic name
Tbsp	Tablespoon	May be confused with tsp (teaspoon)	Write "15 mL"

TABLE 5.1. (*CONTINUED*)

Abbreviation	Intended Meaning	Potential Misinterpretation	Recommendations
Td	Tetanus diphtheria	May be confused with PPD	
TID or tid	Three times daily	May be misinterpreted	Write out "every 8 hours"
Tsp	Teaspoon	May be misinterpreted as tablespoon	Spell out or use "5 mL"
TIW or tiw	3 times a week	May be interpreted as 3 times a day or twice a week	Spell out
U	Unit or units	May be interpreted as O, 4, or CC	Write "unit" or "units"
UD	Units per day	May be interpreted as 60 cc/hr or unit dose	Spell out
$ZnSO_4$	Zinc sulfate	May be confused with ferrous sulfate ($FeSO_4$)	Spell out
Z-PAK	Azithromycin pack	May be read as 2 packs	Write out generic name

Sources: United States Pharmacopeia, 2004a, 2004b.

administration was next at 26 to 38 percent, followed by transcription errors, 11 to 12 percent, and pharmacy dispensing errors, 11 to 14 percent (Bates and others, 1995; Leape and others, 1995).

The following sections look more closely at specific parts of the medication use process.

Prescribing Process Issues: Benefits of an Integrated CPOE System in the Hospital

In paper-based (noncomputerized) prescriber ordering systems, a physician (or other authorized health care provider) writes a medication order in a patient's chart. A clerk may take a copy of that order and fax it to the pharmacy, or put a hard copy of the order in an out-box to be picked up by a pharmacy technician. A nurse will manually transcribe the physician's order onto the patient's medication administration record (MAR), and later a different nurse will probably be the one giving the medication to the patient. The key is to simplify this process and provide less opportunity for error. How? By instituting *computerized prescriber order entry* (CPOE). The patient's name and the drug's name are entered into the CPOE program, and the physician responds to several screen prompts about dosage, duration, and route. Incorrect doses (those not presented as choices) and tenfold dosing errors that occur because a decimal point was not recognized or a capital letter "U" (for *units*) was mistaken for a zero are diminished or eliminated (see JCAHO's 2004 Patient Safety Goal 2b in Exhibit 5.1 and also Table 5.1). Once the computer system approves and finalizes the order, that order simultaneously appears on the patient's MAR and goes to the pharmacy's computer system for review, processing, and dispensing, undergoing a second safety check there for drug interactions and contraindications.

One study indicated that CPOE decreased serious medication errors by 55 percent and reduced potential adverse drug experiences (ADEs) by 84 percent (Bates and others, 1998). These numbers translate directly to dollars. In 1992, Later Day Saints (LDS) Hospital in Salt Lake City had 567 ADEs, which cost the hospital $1.1 million dollars in direct costs (not including the costs of injuries to patients or legal costs). If half of these ADEs had been prevented, LDS Hospital would have saved over $500,000 (Classen and others, 1997). The AHRQ statistics on the effectiveness of instituting advances in reducing medication errors and ADEs are impressive. CPOE saves money and lives (AHRQ, 2001).

AHRQ Findings: ADEs and Costs

- Patients who experience ADEs have longer hospital stays.
- A typical ADE costs $2,000 to 2,500; a preventable ADE costs ~$4,500.
- Additional costs from an ADE range from $1,000 to $2,000 per day.
- Computerized monitoring systems can reduce medication errors by 28 to 95 percent.
- Hospitals can save millions of dollars in direct costs by reducing ADEs.

However, if not carefully and thoughtfully implemented, the use of computers in health care can create new errors:

> *Computer entry* was the fifth leading cause of errors reported to [USP's MEDMARX error reporting program] for both 2000 and 2001 [USP, 2002a, 2002b]. . . . This underscores concerns and cautions raised by researchers and patient safety leaders that if not done carefully, implementation of CPOE and other computer-based programs can result in new errors.
>
> Approximately 10% (35,747/345,600) of all MEDMARX records from September 1998 through December 2002 documented computer entry as a cause of error. Of those, 2% (635 records) indicated the patient was harmed [USP 2003]. In 2001, computer entry was listed as a cause in 11% of all reports where an error did occur ($N = 94,498$) [see Figure 5.3] [USP, 2002b].

As shown in Table 5.2, the most frequently reported types of error associated with computer entry errors were improper dose or quantity, omission error (failure

FIGURE 5.3. TOP TEN CAUSES OF ERROR.

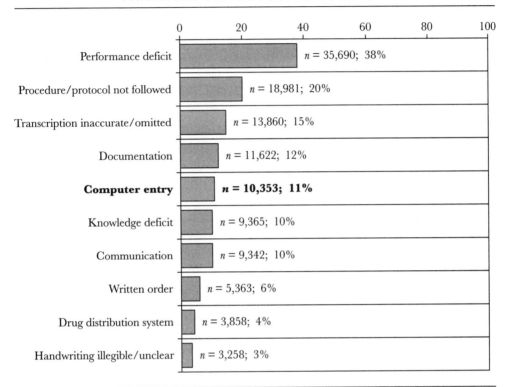

Source: USP, 2002b; based on 94,498 records.

to administer), and prescribing error (owing to drug-drug or drug-food allergies, patient's condition, or an incomplete order).

Reports to MEDMARX reveal the common errors resulting from computer entry (USP, 2003):

- Dosing errors
  Look-alike strengths in close proximity on screen (e.g., 40,000 versus 4,000 units/mL)
  Multiple and differing sliding scales (e.g., potassium, insulin)
  Inadequate dosing algorithms or adjustments for renal failure
- Wrong drug errors
  Numerous similar drug names within single drug class (e.g., insulins)
  Incorrect drug selected for patient's condition or current drug therapy regimen

TABLE 5.2. TYPES OF ERROR ASSOCIATED WITH COMPUTER ENTRY.

Type of Error	n	%
Improper dose/quantity	8,868	28.4
Omission error	6,526	20.9
Prescribing error	5,391	17.2
Unauthorized/wrong drug	3,924	12.5
Wrong time	2,632	8.4
Extra dose	2,513	8
Wrong patient	2,148	6.9
Wrong drug preparation	1,238	4
Wrong dosage form	1,148	3.7
Wrong route	900	2.9
Wrong administration technique	207	0.7
Expired product[a]	4	0.01

Note: Data from MEDMARX records from September 1998 through December 2002 (*N* = 31,272 records).

[a]New type added (2002).

Source: USP, 2003.

- Wrong patient errors
  Incorrect patient selected from screen due to distractions or patients with similar names in same nursing unit (e.g., Smith, Ron vs Smith, Robert) or similar names within an outpatient pharmacy computer information system.

Preventing Computer Entry Errors

USP has disseminated the following general recommendations to reduce errors associated CPOE and other computer entry activities (including CPOE) (USP, 2003):

- Conduct a Failure Mode and Effects Analysis (FMEA) on the use of computers in the various stages of the medication use process to identify potentially confusing abbreviations, dose designations, dosage forms, drug names, and other problems that may be unique to the use of computers to convey information.
- Standardize and simplify all dosing protocols, including sliding scales, to the extent possible prior to implementing CPOE. Take into account complex or unique drug orders (e.g., *"hold 4pm dose until . . . ,"* steroid tapers).
- Allocate ample space in the data fields that are used to communicate patient names, drug names, dosing units, routes of administration, and frequencies. Include properly spaced commas for dose numbers expressed in thousands (e.g., 4,000 units).

- Use USP standard abbreviations for dosage units to express weights and measures in a consistent manner as follows:
  1. m (lower case) = meter
  2. kg = kilogram
  3. g = gram
  4. mg = milligram
  5. mcg = microgram (do not use the Greek letter mu [μ] which has been misread as mg)
  6. L (upper case) = liter
  7. mL (lower/upper case) = milliliter (do not use cc which has been misread as U or the number 4)
  8. mEq = milliequivalent
  9. mmol = millimole.
- Carefully construct the clinical rules/decision support framework using appropriate in-house and outside expertise. The quality of the clinical rules used will have a significant impact on the error-risk potential.
- Establish the proper balance between sensitivity and specificity for computer warnings/alerts to reduce . . . "false-alarm" fatigue [among practitioners] leading to frequent overrides of the warnings.
- Interface CPOE with the medication administration record (MAR) as well as pharmacy and laboratory computer systems to maximize the exchange of accurate and up-to-date patient information.
- Establish a culture among prescribers and other practitioners that creates an openness and willingness to transition to new operational methods for providing health care that uses electronic information technology.

General USP Recommendations for Preventing Prescribing and Transcribing Errors

- Prescribers should submit orders electronically and avoid the need for additional handwritten transcription.
- Prescribers should order or select only standardized concentrations when ordering IV infusions.
- Protocols for ordering IV infusions should be clear and should eliminate the possibility of calculation errors.
- Prescribers should avoid the use of unclear or unsafe abbreviations (Table 5.1).
- Transcription of original orders to medication administration records should be timely, with minimal interruption, and should be independently verified for accuracy. Optimally, transcription should be done electronically, as the manual process (for example, recopying and assigning administration times) is repetitive and has been shown to be error prone (Hicks, Cousins, and Williams, 2003).

Dispensing Process Issues

A medication order goes through numerous processing steps once it reaches the pharmacy. Initially, it should be reviewed by a pharmacist, using clinical rules built into a computer system. This system should evaluate the order against the patient's other prescribed medications for potential drug-drug interactions, contraindications, and inappropriate dose or route based on the patient's age, disease state(s), and clinical condition. If the order is deemed appropriate as written, the pharmacy prepares the medication and delivers it to the nursing unit or patient care area, or ensures that a sufficient quantity exists in the unit's medication storage area or automated dispensing device (for example, Pyxis). Delivery to the floor can be done in many ways. A pharmacist, pharmacy technician, or other designee may bring medications to the floor and place them in a drop-off box, place them in a patient-specific drug drawer, or simply place them in the medication room, cabinet, or automated dispensing machine. Many larger hospitals use automation (for example, pneumatic tubes) to deliver drugs quickly to nursing units spread across their expansive buildings. In addition to having various drug delivery modes, the vast majority of hospitals use a combination of processes for balancing medication supply and demand in the health care facility. The pharmacy may prepare and deliver a single, patient-specific, unit-dose package for some types of orders and for others it may provide a twenty-four-hour supply. Frequently used medications may be stocked routinely on the unit, and nurses may have to go to the medication storage area, medication refrigerator, or automated dispensing machine to retrieve the proper medication for the patient.

Each of these scenarios provides an opportunity for error. The ideal situation is to have the pharmacy dispense all ordered medications in unit-dose form (or as close as possible to it) to minimize the need for further calculation or manipulation by nursing staff. Labeling on unit-dose packages should contain the patient's name, nursing unit, room number, medication name, dose, frequency of administration, and route of administration (Hicks, Cousins, and Williams, 2003).

General USP Recommendations for Preventing Dispensing Errors

- Pharmacy services should stock or prepare standardized concentrations for all IV medications. Intravenous solution bags should be properly labeled with the complete patient name and should display the product(s) or ingredient(s) name, the dosage(s), the final concentration of the product(s), and the infusion rate, as appropriate.
- Commercially prepared solutions should be used whenever possible. Use of different strengths of the same solution or medication in a facility should be limited and standardized.

- The pharmacy should always dispense a unit-of-use (as opposed to a multidose) package, to the extent possible, to avert the potential for improper dose or quantity errors (Hicks, Cousins, and Williams, 2003).

Administering and Monitoring Medication

According to data from USP's 2002 MEDMARX data summary report (Hicks, Cousins, and Williams, 2003), approximately one-third of reported errors occur in the administering stage of the medication use process and 1 percent in the monitoring stage. *Wrong-patient* errors rank seventh in frequency among the fourteen different types of error. With a computerized *bar-coding* system, both the patient's and medication's identification can be incorporated into the medication label. If the patient wears a bar-coded identification bracelet, then the patient also can be identified more easily, and facilities will move halfway toward satisfying the JCAHO's first Patient Safety Goal for 2004—"Improve the accuracy of patient identification"—by using "at least two patient identifiers . . . whenever administering medications or blood" (see Exhibit 5.1). Both the FDA and the NCC MERP agree that placing bar codes on drug packaging can improve patient safety (FDA, 2004). Since 1999, Veterans Administration (VA) hospitals have employed the VA Bar Code Administration Project (BCAP), which has prevented an estimated 378,000 medication errors (Cannistra, 2002). The FDA estimates that bar coding could save hospitals $41.4 billion in direct costs and an additional $7.6 billion in administrative costs by preventing 50 percent of their medication errors (Becker, 2003).

General USP Recommendations for Preventing Administering and Monitoring Errors

- Staff should be familiar with the institution's policies and procedures for medication administration.
- Preprinted and standardized infusion rate charts should be readily accessible and widely used. These charts offer some protection against calculation errors.
- Programmable infusion devices (for example, *smart pumps*) that offer customized settings to meet the hospital's guidelines for selected drug dosages for specific patient types and specialized clinical care areas should be widely used. Variability of types and models of infusion devices should be limited to avoid staff confusion.
- Infusion pump settings for initiation of high-alert medications *and* for any required dosage adjustment should be independently confirmed by two qualified individuals.
- Documentation of the medication infusion, adjustments, and independent confirmation should be readily apparent.

- Infusion tubing should be traced from the infusion bag to the point of delivery (where it reaches the patient). If multiple infusions and pumps are in use on a patient, each pump and its respective tubing should be readily identifiable and labeled.
- Free-flow errors can be avoided through proper and reasonable safety measures. IV administration cassettes that offer anti-free-flow mechanisms should be used routinely. Free flow should be avoided when the IV administration cassette has been removed from the pump (that is, during a gown change or to clear air).
- The patient's clinical response to the medication infusion should be monitored according to critical pathways that incorporate standardized flow sheets or monitoring protocols developed by interdisciplinary committees. The therapeutic class of the medication, particularly of high-alert drugs, should dictate the type of observation (for example, cardiopulmonary function or laboratory values) (Hicks, Cousins, and Williams, 2003).

Medication Errors That Do Not Reach or Cause Harm to a Patient

Some individuals use the term *near miss* to refer to a medication error that did not reach the patient or to describe a system that failed but did not cause harm to the patient. However, despite the fact that the patient was not injured, an error did occur. That error was a signal that the system is not error-proof and needs to be fixed. Excluding a near miss from an analysis of medication errors simply because a patient was not injured prevents the risk management team from learning valuable information about the system or process that failed. This information about near misses can be acted on to minimize or prevent the recurrence of similar system failure–induced medication errors (Cohoon, 2003).

The Joint Commission on Accreditation of Healthcare Organizations recognizes the value of identifying and analyzing near misses in its definition of a reportable *sentinel event* as "an unexpected occurrence involving death or serious physical or psychological injury, or the risk thereof." "Risk thereof" means that this definition includes "any process variation for which a recurrence would carry a significant chance of serious adverse outcome" (JCAHO, 2002), indicating that if the process or system isn't reengineered, another error is likely to occur. Remember, those who misread history are doomed to repeat the mistakes of the past!

Types of Drugs Most Commonly Involved in Medication Errors

JCAHO's Sentinel Event Program has identified the following high-alert drugs (JCAHO, 1999).

TABLE 5.3. PRODUCT GROUPS CAUSING PATIENT HARM MOST COMMONLY REPORTED TO MEDMARX.

	Product's Generic Name	*n*	%
Errors involving harm (Categories E–I)	Insulin[a]	244	8.1
	Morphine[a]	164	5.5
	Heparin[a]	139	4.6
	Potassium Chloride[a]	90	3.0
	Warfarin[a]	89	3.0
	Hydromorphone[a]	83	2.8
	Fentanyl[a]	66	2.2
	Vancomycin	61	2.0
	Enoxaparin	60	2.0
	Meperidine[a]	57	1.9
	Furosemide	52	1.7
	Diltiazem	45	1.5
	Metoprolol	38	1.3
	Dopamine	37	1.2
	Lorazepam	37	1.2

Note: Product groups include all dosage forms and formulations.

[a]High-alert medication.

Source: Hicks, Cousins, and Williams, 2003.

High-Alert Drugs Identified by JCAHO

- Concentrated electrolytes including KCl, Potassium phosphate, and NaCl (>0.9 percent)
- Insulin
- Opiates, narcotics, and patient controlled analgesia (PCA)
- IV anticoagulants, such as Heparin

USP's MEDMARX program has identified a similar list of high-alert drugs, summarized in Table 5.3. In addition a recent study (Benjamin and Pendrak, 2003) has summarized the drugs most frequently cited in the PHICO Insurance Company's Closed Claims project:

Drugs Involved in Claims at PHICO: Two out of Three Years Between 1996 and 1998.

- Antibiotics
- Electrolytes
- Opiates
- Anticoagulants
- Tranquilizers

TABLE 5.4. TYPES OF MEDICATION ERRORS TRIGGERING CLAIMS IN 1998.

Type of Error	%
Allergic/adverse reaction	25
Contraindicated drug given	22
IM technique issue	10
Wrong dose	10
Wrong drug	10
Wrong patient	3
Wrong route	3
Labeling/dispensing error	1
Not classified, includes failure to monitor & failure to prescribe	17

Source: Data from Benjamin and Pendrak, 2003.

- Fibrinolytics
- Insulin
- Oral antidiabetics
- Antihypertensives

The PHICO data also captured the types of medication errors that triggered claims. It is apparent from these data (Table 5.4) that the same basic medication errors (sometimes called the *five wrongs*) continue to be made: wrong drug, wrong dose, wrong time, wrong route, and wrong patient. Inadequate monitoring or failure to follow up can also lead to adverse drug reactions. However, first on PHICO's list is allergic or adverse reaction, which constituted 25 percent of medication error claims, meaning that patients who were allergic to a drug or had a history of not tolerating a drug well received the same drug again. Second on the list is contraindicated drug, with 22 percent of claims due to that problem. A drug is contraindicated when the patient has a peculiar sensitivity to it, when the patient is taking other medications that can interact with the proposed drug and increase its toxicity or decrease its effectiveness, when the patient is pregnant or nursing and should not receive the drug because of maternal-fetal or maternal-infant transmission, or when the patient has some pathological condition (for example, decreased renal or hepatic function) that makes the drug more toxic in that patient. Usually no strict contraindication exists for using drugs in patients with decreased renal or hepatic function, but the dose must be greatly reduced. In the reported claims, significant injury must have occurred or the patient would not have had sufficient damages to sustain a lawsuit. Drug-drug interactions have also been the primary cause of the withdrawal from the market of many well-known drugs, such as Seldane (terfenadine), Hismanyl (astemizole), Posicor (mibefradil), and Propulsid (cisapride) (Benjamin, 2001a). Had CPOE been available, the computer could have alerted prescribers to the potential drug-drug interactions, dosages could have been reduced, and both nationwide drug recalls and patient injury could have been averted.

Medication Errors and Human Factors

People make errors. It is part of being human. Mental errors can occur during periods of high stress—when the nursing unit or patient care area is understaffed or the workload is unrealistically high—or they can occur when people are distracted—by a phone call, page, banter, or ordering pizza. However, the people we work with are not only staff, they are our colleagues and friends, and now more than ever, health care is truly a team effort. The physician is the head of the team but needs assistance and feedback from all team members in order to establish and maintain the needed culture of patient safety. Each member of the team should collaborate with other members to establish a safety net designed to catch errors and to identify system flaws (practices) that can lead to errors so these flaws can be rectified before errors occur. Because of the large number of people and professions employed in the institutional setting, professionals who supervise other employees are responsible for reviewing their work and ensuring that they are adequately trained and performing at an acceptable level. Pharmacists should check medications prepared and dispensed by technicians before they are delivered to nursing units or floor stock or placed in automated dispensing devices. Nurses should care for sicker patients and let nursing assistants care for patients who do not need to be monitored as closely. No one should program an IV pump, PCA machine, or other piece of equipment unless he or she is well educated about the equipment (see JCAHO's 2004 Patient Safety Goal 5 in Exhibit 5.1). The American Society for Healthcare Risk Management (ASHRM) discusses many aspects of human factors in medication error reduction and reviews much of the recent medication error literature in its publication *Risk Management PEARLS for Medication Error Reduction* (Benjamin and others, 2001).

Defining Medication Error

The National Coordinating Council for Medication Error Reporting and Prevention (NCC MERP) was established in 1995 and includes representation from the U.S. Pharmacopeia, FDA, JCAHO, Institute for Safe Medical Practices (ISMP), American Hospital Association (AHA), American Medical Association (AMA), American Nursing Association (ANA), American Society for Healthcare

Risk Management (ASHRM), and American Society of Health-System Pharmacists (ASHP). NCC MERP has developed a comprehensive medication error taxonomy and definition that has come to be widely recognized and accepted by health care professionals. The council defines a medication error as "any preventable event that may cause or lead to inappropriate medication use or patient harm while the medication is in the control of the healthcare professional, patient, or consumer. Such events may be related to professional practice, healthcare products, procedures, and systems, including prescribing; order communication; product labeling, packaging, and nomenclature; compounding; dispensing; distribution; administration; education; monitoring; and use" (NCC MERP, 2004). Of course, the most important word in the definition is *preventable*.

What Small Facilities with Limited Resources Can Do to Prevent Medication Errors

The first thing for small facilities to do when they cannot afford to computerize or adopt other innovative technology is to review the lists of high-risk drugs and common medication errors given in this chapter. This is an important starting place. All of these drugs can cause serious injury or death to patients. In order to reduce the likelihood of patient injury, prepare a memorandum containing the names and classes of these drugs and circulate the memo to physicians, pharmacists, and nurses in your facility. Announce to your staff that these are the drugs that can cause the most harm and that staff should be cautious and vigilant when prescribing, dispensing, or administering them to patients.

To eliminate the risk of excessive doses, consider developing special protocols or standardized order forms for high-risk drugs that list the lowest or most common doses, frequencies, and routes of administration. Such preprinted order forms allow the prescriber to simply check off the desired prescription requirements for the patient. Also include known drug-drug interactions and clinical conditions and contraindications that need to be ruled out prior to initiation of therapy. Remember also that the drugs listed in this chapter are not the only drugs that can cause unintended injury to a patient. Aminoglycoside antibiotics and digoxin must be given at lower doses to patients with renal failure to avoid toxicity. Antihypertensives, tricyclic antidepressants, alpha-blockers (now used to facilitate urination in patients with benign prostatic hyperplasia), and narcotics all can cause fainting or orthostatic (positional) hypotension and lead to falls in the hospital and at home.

Problems with ordering drugs can be ameliorated by implementing a training program for your prescribers. An excellent and free resource for training prescribers can be found on the Tufts University School of Medicine Web site. This Web-based teaching program, titled "Prescription Writing: A Mini Learning Module" (Shader and Benjamin, 2001), has been used to retrain physicians who have lost their prescribing privileges, medical students, nurse practitioners, and physician assistants. The course also offers a review of abbreviations, acronyms, and symbols that should and should not be used in writing prescriptions and provides guidance on how to write a prescription or drug order that communicates the desired information in the most effective, least ambiguous way, as recommended in JCAHO's 2004 Patient Safety Goal 2b (see Exhibit 5.1 and Table 5.1).

In addition to identifying faulty processes and potential system failures, health care facilities must also update their philosophies for dealing with people and events that have led or could lead to medication errors. Contemporary experts in reducing medication errors all stress developing a *culture of safety* and dispensing with the anachronistic practice of finding someone to blame. Today's objectives are to identify high-risk practices and failure-prone areas of the medication use process and then *fix* them! When a medication error occurs, do a *root cause analysis* (RCA), not because JCAHO requires it of accredited hospitals but in order to figure out *why* the error occurred. Hold monthly quality improvement meetings, and review the RCA results with staff. Also ask members of the medical, nursing, and pharmacy staffs to bring areas of concern to the attention of the rest of the staff. You may want to begin by having medicine, pharmacy, and nursing personnel meet separately and then bring the entire group together after everyone is comfortable with the process.

Several years ago, one of the authors of this chapter (DMB) was asked to conduct a risk management audit of a large Midwestern hospital that had experienced ten respiratory depressions (and two deaths) over the past two years in patients receiving patient controlled analgesia. During the course of the site visit, he asked the hospital risk manager if she ever got the doctors, the pharmacists, and the nurses together to talk about any concerns any of them had regarding medication ordering, dispensing, or administration. The answer was no. He recommended that the risk management practitioner function establish such a committee. About a year later, the nurse risk manager called him to tell him she had been accepted to law school and also mentioned that she had established a committee of doctors, pharmacists, and nurses to discuss medication errors. She also said that as a result of some of his specific recommendations for reducing the concomitant use of narcotics, Benadryl, hydroxyzine, Phenergan, and a benzodiazepine "sleeping pill" in the same patient and his urging to "bring everything out in the open" under the peer review function of the hospital, there had been no further respiratory depressions (or deaths) in the last year. The lesson to be learned is, if you don't identify the problem, analyze the problem, and take steps to change those areas that lead to patient injury, you can't prevent that problem from occurring again.

Be very selective about adding new drugs to the hospital formulary. Newly approved drugs have been tested in only approximately 5,000 patients. Safety data about rare but severe adverse drug reactions like Stevens-Johnson syndrome, toxic epidermal necrolysis (TEN), and acute renal failure may not have been reported or included in the labeling (package insert), and these reactions could occur even though you don't anticipate them (Benjamin, 1998). For this reason, it is also important to review a product's labeling every year to determine whether new warnings have been added because of postmarketing reports of adverse drug reactions.

Lastly, review JCAHO's current National Patient Safety Goals (NPSGs) (for example, Exhibit 5.1) and implement as many goals (or acceptable alternatives) as possible, whether your organization is a JCAHO-accredited facility or not. Why? Because these patient safety goals were developed after reviewing actual instances of medication errors, are evidence based, and will assist your facility in improving quality of care, reducing medication errors, and increasing patient safety.

Medication Error Reduction in the Outpatient Setting

When it comes to prescribing drugs for patients, most clinical pharmacologists are *therapeutic nihilists*. It follows logically that if you don't want to have to treat any adverse drug reactions in your patients, then don't prescribe any drugs for them. However, if you really must prescribe drugs, use the lowest dose, for the shortest time. Moreover, the likelihood of a drug-drug interaction increases as more drugs are added to the patient's regimen. In order to reduce the likelihood of drug-drug interactions, and also the additive effects of similarly acting medications, prescribe as few drugs as possible, at the lowest dose, for the shortest period of time. Whenever possible, prescribe something for topical or local use rather than a systemic medication. When you write an initial prescription, order only one to two weeks worth of medication. Many patients discontinue their medications, can't tolerate them, or switch to another drug prior to using all the medication or dosing strength originally prescribed. The adage "Start low—go slow" remains valid.

In 1982, the National Council on Patient Information and Education (NCPIE) was formed to raise awareness about the role of communication in promoting safe, appropriate use of medications. NCPIE (2004) offers some very useful information about U.S. physicians' prescribing practices. For example, in 1998, nearly two-thirds (65.1 percent) of physician office visits culminated with the writing of a prescription, 36.5 percent of patients received two or more prescriptions, and over 10 percent received four or more prescriptions. Over 80 percent of office visits to cardiologists resulted in a prescription, although only 18 percent of visits to general surgeons did so. In 2000, there were 2.7 billion retail prescriptions filled, which brought in revenues of $148.2 billion; in 2001, 3.3 billion were filled, which cost $175.2 billion; and by 2004, the number of retail prescriptions is expected to exceed 4 billion, and an even greater amount of resources will be spent.

Problems Contributing to Medication Errors in the Outpatient Setting

From the NCPIE data, it is obvious that physicians are prescribing drugs too often and that polypharmacotherapy is rampant. Moreover, a recent report from the Institute of Medicine (2003) concluded that health professionals are not being adequately prepared to provide the highest-quality and safest medical care possible and that there is insufficient assessment of their ongoing proficiency. Indeed, another recent study of formal training on medication errors in medical school indicates that only 16 percent of internal medicine clerkships include formal lectures on adverse drug reactions and drug-drug interactions (Rosebraugh and others, 2001). The message is clear. More teaching has to be done in this area. Also, physicians apparently need to adjust the way they view medical error. Despite the fact that 35 percent of physicians surveyed reported errors in their own care or the care of a family member, medical error was not considered one of the greatest problems in health care today. Instead, physicians emphasized the cost of malpractice insurance and lawsuits (29 percent), the cost of health care (27 percent), and problems with insurance companies and health plans (22 percent). Only 5 percent of physicians identified medical errors as one of the most serious problems (Blendon and others, 2002).

Although the costs of obtaining malpractice insurance are high (especially for certain high-risk specialties), physicians and others who believe that lawsuits are the greatest impediment to quality health care are not only mistaken but are ten years behind in reading the literature, as indicated by the famous Harvard Medical Practice Study (Localio and others, 1991). As part of this landmark study, investigators reviewed approximately 31,000 charts for evidence of malpractice and found 280 instances of medical negligence. However, only 8 of the 280 instances of malpractice resulted in lawsuits, an incidence of less than 3 percent. The authors correctly concluded that patients who deserved to be compensated for negligence had not been compensated. In these cases, negligence was identified rarely, and providers of substandard care rarely were held accountable for their actions. In actuality, the major reasons patients sue their doctors are poor communication and problematic relationships (Beckman, Markakis, Suchman, and Frankel, 1994). Some of the reasons cited in Beckman and others' review of forty-five plaintiffs' depositions are that the patient felt deserted by the doctor (32 percent), the patient felt the doctor devalued the patient's or a family member's view or perspective (42 percent), and the doctor delivered information poorly (26 percent). Many other studies have come to the same conclusion. For example, another decade-old study (Hickson and others, 1994) concluded that patients of physicians who had been sued frequently had more complaints about the interpersonal care and physician-patient communication the doctors provided than did patients of doctors who had not been sued repeatedly. Some of the complaints were that patients felt rushed, test results were not explained, and the patients felt ignored. The lesson to be learned is that if you are a physician who wants to reduce your exposure to a lawsuit, your communication skills are more important than your clinical skills. Patients won't sue you if they like you.

It would seem that physicians are not willing to take responsibility for their own actions and that they are more willing to blame insurance companies and lawsuits than they are willing to stay current in their fields. This type of hubris will only perpetuate the communication and education deficit in health care today, not ameliorate it. According to a recent study from the RAND Corporation, a corporate think tank, patients received the "recommended care" for thirty common acute and chronic conditions only about 55.5 percent of the time. In an interview published in the *Washington Post,* the study's lead author, Elizabeth A. McGlynn, said, "Everyone is at risk of failing to get care that they need to live a longer and healthier life. . . . It is time to stop having a debate whether we have a problem, and start having a talk about how we can solve the problem" (Brown, 2003, p. A02).

Some problems arising from the apparently low quality of care provided and the misuse of medications can be cured by continuing education and the expanding role of information technology. For example, another landmark study identified the major system errors responsible for medication errors that resulted in adverse drug events. Lack of knowledge about the drug and lack of information about the patient were major contributing factors. The authors concluded that "the most common defects were in systems to disseminate knowledge about drugs and to make drug and patient information readily accessible at the time it is needed" (Leape and others, 1995, p. 35). Certainly CPOE and electronic medical records could be instrumental in decreasing errors caused by deficits in knowledge about either the drug or the patient. Now do we all accept that we can't keep all the information in our heads that we need to practice our professions?

Although the process for writing and dispensing a prescription in the outpatient setting is a lot less complicated than it is in an institutional setting, many of the same problems arise. A poorly written prescription is still a poorly written prescription. At the least it means that the pharmacist will have to call the physician for clarification. At the worst the pharmacist guesses, and a medication error may well be made.

Decreasing Dispensing Errors in the Outpatient Setting

Outpatient pharmacies still stock drugs alphabetically, and look-alike drugs may be found right next to each other. Sometimes there is confusion between a *regular-acting* formulation—say, for a drug like theophylline (for asthma)—and a *sustained-release* (SR) formulation. Sometimes the wrong dose is dispensed for the right drug.

Using computerized bar codes, based on each drug's NDC number, is a good way to minimize or eliminate wrong-dose or wrong-formulation dispensing errors.

Telephone orders present another type of problem. Imagine how easily Cardiem and Cardizem can be confused when a doctor calls in a prescription to a pharmacy. Or better yet, how about the difficulty of distinguishing verbal orders for Celebrex, Cerebryx, and Celexa? The proper procedure for calling in a prescription is for the doctor to dictate the prescription order as the pharmacist writes it down. Then the pharmacist must *read back* the order, just as it was transcribed. This could be the last chance to at least record the prescription order properly. Getting the right drug off the shelf and putting it in the right container and labeling the container with the right directions still provide plenty of opportunities for error. What all health care providers are trying to achieve is referred to collectively as *the five rights:* the right drug, the right dose, the right route, the right time, and the right patient!

Conclusion: The Imperative for Federal Legislation

Since the publication of the Institute of Medicine report *To Err Is Human: Building a Safer Health System* (Kohn, Corrigan, and Donaldson, 2000), awareness of medication errors has been elevated to the national level. In an effort to improve the quality of health care and reduce medical errors, numerous federal bills have been introduced to encourage medication error reporting and quality improvement initiatives. Although no federal bill has been enacted, it appears that Congress has made tremendous progress toward adopting legislation that would provide protection (create a federal privilege) for patient safety data, including medication error reports.

In response to the IOM report, Congress has been working toward implementing federal patient safety legislation. Recommendation 6.1. of the IOM report encourages Congress to pass legislation that creates a legal environment that encourages "health care professionals and organizations to identify, analyze, and prevent errors without increasing the threat of litigation and without compromising patients' rights" (Kohn, Corrigan, and Donaldson, 2000, p. 96). The IOM report recognizes that no federal protection currently exists against the disclosure of medication error information that is shared with reporting programs for health care facilities and practitioners. Absent clear federal legal protection, practitioners will continue to resist requests to report medication errors in a consistent and uniform manner, a situation that merely mimics the status quo and perpetuates our current inability to recognize and identify many medication errors. The continued lack of privilege also impairs the efforts of educators and

researchers to improve the quality of pharmacotherapy at the national level, now
and in the future.

During the 107th Congress (January 2001 to December 2002) five medical
error reporting bills were introduced but not passed, including S 3029, sponsored
by Senator Kennedy; S 2390, sponsored by Senators Frist and Jeffords; HR 4889,
sponsored by Representative Johnson; and HR 5478, introduced by Representative Bilirakis. These bills proposed to encourage medical and medication error
reporting by establishing a federal privilege for information submitted to patient
safety reporting programs (commonly referred to in the bills as *patient safety organizations* [PSOs]). Such legislation would build on the foundations of a similar standard adopted by the state of Oklahoma on May 8, 2001, which provides that
reports to the U.S. Pharmacopeia's MEDMARX system are to be considered privileged communications and cannot be introduced as evidence in any legal proceeding (Benjamin and others, 2001). Although progress was made toward
implementing patient safety legislation during the 107th Congress, important differences among the bills were not resolved. These differences involved the extent
of legal privilege and confidentiality and the qualification of PSOs.

In January 2003, the 108th Congress began, and patient safety legislation was
once again addressed. On March 12, 2003, the House of Representatives passed
the Patient Safety and Quality Improvement Act (HR 663) to encourage the
voluntary reporting and analysis of medication errors. Section 2(b) of HR 663
was intended to encourage a culture of safety and quality by providing for a
reporting system that both protected information and improved patient safety, thus
improving the quality of health care. On March 26, 2003, Senators Gregg, Frist,
Jeffords, and Breaux reintroduced the patient safety legislation (S 720) first introduced in the Senate during the 107th Congress. The bill was revised, and on
July 23, 2003, the Senate Health, Education, Labor, and Pensions (HELP) Committee unanimously approved the revised legislation. According to Section 2(b) of
the Act, the purpose of S 720 is "to encourage a culture of safety and quality by
providing for legal protection of information reported voluntarily for the purposes
of quality improvement and patient safety." The Senate had hoped to vote on the
legislation by the end of the year.

Although federal patient safety legislation has yet to pass both the House and
Senate, it appears that Congress is well positioned to accomplish this goal. Federal
protection for patient safety data, including medication error reports shared with
PSOs, should help to reduce medication errors, increase the quality of pharmaceutical care, and improve patient safety in the United States. Failure to pass
such legislation would continue to act as a significant obstacle to the full implementation of medication error reporting programs and to the valuable lessons
that can be learned from the examination of reported errors. Without such

legislation, health care facilities and practitioners will continue to be reluctant to track, report, and learn from prior medication errors, thereby reducing opportunities to identify and prevent medication errors at the regional, state, and national level.

There can be no doubt that quality improvement costs a lot less than making errors and defending lawsuits. At an approximate cost of $4,500 per preventable medication error, preventing just twenty-five medication errors saves $112,500. That's enough to hire a PharmD to make rounds in one's intensive care unit (ICU), which can save an additional $270,000 in costs associated with extended hospitalization and costs of additional treatment (excluding the costs of litigation) (Leape and others, 1997; Bates and others, 1998). Moreover, isn't it better to pay for progress and an improved quality of care than to pay to defend a lawsuit that could have been prevented? Those who misread history are doomed to repeat the mistakes of the past. Welcome to the era of enlightenment. The tools of progress are available to us right now. What are we going to do with them, build a better health care system or hit our thumbs with the hammer?

References

Agency for Healthcare Research and Quality. "Reducing and Preventing Adverse Drug Events to Decrease Hospital Costs." *Research in Action,* Issue 1. [http://www.ahrq.gov/qual/aderia/aderia.htm]. Mar. 2001.

Bates, D. W., and others. "Incidence of Adverse Drug Events and Potential Adverse Drug Events." *Journal of the American Medical Association,* 1995, *274,* 29–34.

Bates, D. W., and others. "Effect of Computerized Physician Order Entry and a Team Intervention on Prevention of Serious Medication Errors." *Journal of the American Medical Association,* 1998, *280,* 1311–1316.

Becker C. "Scanning for Higher Profits." *Modern Healthcare,* June 16, 2003.

Beckman, H. B., Markakis, K. M., Suchman, A. L., and Frankel, R. M. "The Doctor-Patient Relationship and Malpractice." *Archives of Internal Medicine,* 1994, *154,* 1365–1370.

Benjamin, D. M. "Pharmaceutical Risk Management: Special Problems Encountered in the Hospital Setting." *Journal of Healthcare Risk Management,* 1998, *18,* 5–17.

Benjamin, D. M. "Drug Approvals, Drug Withdrawals: 'Déjà Vu All Over Again.'" *Pharmaceutical & Medical Device Law Bulletin,* 2001a, *1,* 3–5.

Benjamin, D. M. "Reducing Medication Errors and Increasing Patient Safety Through Better Communication." *Focus on Patient Safety* (National Patient Safety Foundation), 2001b, *4*(6, 8).

Benjamin, D. M., and others. "Risk Management PEARLS for Medication Error Reduction." *Journal of Healthcare Risk Management,* 2001, pp. 41–52.

Benjamin, D. M., and Pendrak, R. F. "Medication Errors: An Analysis Comparing PHICO's Closed Claims Data and PHICO's Event Reporting Trending System (PERTS)." *Journal of Clinical Pharmacology,* 2003, *43,* 754–759.

Blendon, R. J., and others. "Patient Safety: Views of Practicing Physicians and the Public on Medical Errors." *New England Journal of Medicine,* 2002, *347,* 1933–1940.

Brown, D. "Medical Care Often Not Optimal, Study Finds." *Washington Post,* June 26, 2003, p. A02.

Cannistra, J. "Bar Code Project Eliminates Medication Errors." *Pharmacy Today,* Aug. 27, 2002, p. 27.

Classen, D. C., and others. "Adverse Drug Events in Hospitalized Patients." *Journal of the American Medical Association,* 1997, *277,* 301–306.

Cohoon, B. D. "Learning from Near Misses Through Reflection: A New Risk Management Strategy." *Journal of Healthcare Risk Management,* 2003, *23,* 19–25.

Coiera, E. "When Conversation Is Better Than Computation." *Journal of the American Medical Informatics Association,* 2000, *7,* 277–286.

ECRI. *HRC Risk Analysis.* Vol. 4. Plymouth Meeting, Penn.: ECRI, 2000.

Food and Drug Administration. "FDA Issues Bar Code Regulation." [http://www.fda.gov/oc/initiatives/barcode-sadr/fs-barcode.html]. Feb. 25, 2004.

Hicks, R. W., Cousins, D. D., and Williams, R. L. *Summary of Information Submitted to MEDMARX^{SM} in the Year 2002: The Quest for Quality.* Rockville, Md.: USP Center for the Advancement of Patient Safety, 2003.

Hickson, G. B., and others. "Obstetricians' Prior Malpractice Experience and Patients' Satisfaction with Care." *Journal of the American Medical Association,* 1994, *272,* 1583–1587.

Institute of Medicine. *Health Professions Education: A Bridge to Quality.* Washington, D.C.: National Academies Press, Apr. 2003.

Joint Commission on Accreditation of Healthcare Organizations. *Sentinel Event Alert,* Nov. 19, 1999, Issue 11.

Joint Commission on Accreditation of Healthcare Organizations. "Hospitals: Sentinel Event Policy and Procedures Revised: July 2002." [http://www.jcaho.org/accredited+organizations/hospitals/sentinel+events/index.htm]. 2002.

Joint Commission on Accreditation of Healthcare Organizations. "2004 National Patient Safety Goals." [http://www.jcaho.org/accredited+organizations/patient+safety/npsg.htm]. 2004.

Kohn, L. T., Corrigan, J. M., and Donaldson, M. S. (eds.). *To Err Is Human: Building a Safer Health System.* Washington, D.C.: National Academies Press, 2000.

Leape, L. L., and others. "Systems Analysis of Adverse Drug Events." *Journal of the American Medical Association,* 1995, *274,* 35–43.

Leape, L. L., and others. "Pharmacist Participation on Physician Rounds and Adverse Drug Events in the Intensive Care Unit." *Journal of the American Medical Association,* 1997, *282,* 267–270.

Leape, L .L., and others. "Promoting Patient Safety by Preventing Medical Error." *Journal of the American Medical Association,* 1998, *280,* 1444.

Localio, A. R., and others. "Relation Between Malpractice Claims and Adverse Events Due to Negligence: Results of the Harvard Medical Practice Study III." *New England Journal of Medicine,* 1991, *325,* 245–251.

National Coordinating Council for Medication Error Reporting and Prevention. "About Medication Errors: Types of Medication Errors." [http://www.nccmerp.org/medError-CatIndex.html]. 2001.

National Coordinating Council for Medication Error Reporting and Prevention. "About Medication Errors." [http://www.nccmerp.org/aboutMedErrors.html]. 2004.

National Council on Patient Information and Education. [www.talkaboutrx.org]. 2004.

Rosebraugh, C. J., and others. "Formal Education About Medication Errors in Internal Medicine Clerkships." *Journal of the American Medical Association*, 2001, *286*, 1019–1020.

Santell, J. P., Hicks, R. W., McMeekin, J., and Cousins, D. D. "Medication Errors: Experience of the United States Pharmacopeia (USP) MEDMARX Reporting System." *Journal of Clinical Pharmacology*, 2003, *43*, 760–767.

Shader, R. I., and Benjamin, D. M. "Prescription Writing: A Mini Learning Module." [http://www.tufts.edu/med/curriculum/prescription_writing.html]. 2001.

United States Pharmacopeia. "Use Caution—Avoid Confusion." *USP Quality Review* (newsletter), Mar. 2001, *76*.

United States Pharmacopeia. *Summary of Information Submitted to MEDMARX^{SM} in the Year 2000: Charting a Course for Change.* Rockville, Md.: United States Pharmacopeia, 2002a.

United States Pharmacopeia. *Summary of Information Submitted to MEDMARX^{SM} in the Year 2001: A Human Factors Approach to Understanding Medication Errors.* Rockville, Md.: United States Pharmacopeia, 2002b.

United States Pharmacopeia, Center for the Advancement of Patient Safety. "USP Patient Safety CAPSLink . . . Risk of Computer Entry Errors and Recommendations for Prevention." [http://www.usp.org/pdf/patientsafety/capsLink2003-05-01.pdf]. May 2003.

United States Pharmacopeia, Center for the Advancement of Patient Safety. "Patient Safety: USP Quality Review: Potentially Dangerous Drug Name Abbreviations." Table 1. [http://www.usp.org/patientSafety/briefsArticlesReports/qualityReview/qr802004-07-01a.html]. July 2004a.

United States Pharmacopeia, Center for the Advancement of Patient Safety. "Patient Safety: USP Quality Review: Potentially Dangerous Abbreviations." Table 2. [http://www.usp.org/patientSafety/briefsArticlesReports/qualityReview/qr802004-07-01b.html] July 2004b.

CHAPTER SIX

BENCHMARKING

Evidence-Based Outcome Information and Standards of Care

Peter J. Pronovost
Fay A. Rozovsky

Health care is striving to become more evidence based. Patients, providers, insurers, regulators, accreditors, and purchasers are all demanding evidence to support improved quality of care. This is warranted. The evidence suggests that much of the morbidity, mortality, and cost of care can be reduced. Although the use of evidence to guide health policy is relatively new, it is likely to increase. Indeed, several groups, including the Centers for Medicare & Medicaid Services (CMS), the National Quality Forum (NQF), and the Joint Commission on Accreditation of Healthcare Organizations (JCAHO), are collaborating to develop measures of quality of care.

How the use of outcome data will inform policy and purchasing decisions is unknown. In this chapter we present an overview of the use of benchmark data for patient safety and then explore how payors, providers, and consumers are using benchmark data. In addition, we discuss whether benchmarking creates a standard of care, and the risks and potential benefits of using benchmark data to create a standard of care.

Benchmarking for Patient Safety: The Use of Evidence-Based Outcome Data

Benchmarking is simply a method of comparing your performance to someone else's. In *internal benchmarking* you compare your performance against prior performance. In *external benchmarking* you compare your performance to that of an outside organization or to some other external standard. Benchmarks generally take the form of measures of quality and are based on the premise that to improve, we need feedback regarding our performance. These measures may be empiric measures of quality, such as the JCAHO performance measures (for example, giving beta-blockers to a patient with a myocardial infarction), or standards such as the JCAHO (2004) safety standards.

More than thirty years ago, Donabedian (1966) proposed that we can measure the quality of health care by observing its structure, its processes, and its outcomes. The Institute of Medicine (IOM) has defined health care quality as "the degree to which health services for individuals and populations increase the likelihood of desired health outcomes and are consistent with current professional knowledge" (Lohr and Schroeder, 1990). The IOM's definition and framework thus incorporate two of Donabedian's three elements in a broad approach to measuring health care quality: (1) determining effects of health care on desired outcomes, including a relative improvement in health and in consumer evaluations or experiences of health care, and (2) assessing the degree to which health care adheres to processes that have been proven by scientific evidence or agreed by professional consensus to affect health or that concur with patient preference.

Measures of quality provide insights into many aspects of quality. For example, one of the authors (PSP) saw something like this occurring when his five-year-old son, Ethan, was asked to make a collage of himself. We pasted into the collage pictures of Ethan with his sister and parents, at the beach, at camp, and at school. Although no single picture allowed the viewer to know Ethan completely, by viewing all the pictures, one could begin to know him. Some of the pictures were clear; others were granular; some were important to Ethan; others were important to his parents, his grandparents, and teachers. Quality measures, like the pictures in a collage, give us many views of the quality of whatever we are trying to learn about.

The IOM has further suggested that health care should have the six aims of being effective, safe, patient-centered, timely, efficient, and equitable (Institute of Medicine, 2001). Whereas the aims of effectiveness and safety in health care are nearly universal, societies and cultures around the world differ in how much emphasis they give to each of the additional aims of patient-centeredness, timeliness, efficiency, and equity. *Process of care* measures of quality assess whether providers perform health care processes that have been demonstrated to achieve the desired aims and avoid those processes that predispose toward harm.

Varied audiences need health care quality measures in order to receive feedback on the quality of care provided. Organizations may use this feedback as they go about health care purchasing, utilization, regulatory accreditation and monitoring, or performance improvement (Pronovost and others, 2004; Rubin, Pronovost, and Diette, 2001). For all these purposes it is imperative that the results of quality measures be meaningful, scientifically sound, generalizable, and interpretable (McGlynn, 1998). To achieve these goals, quality measures must be designed and implemented with scientific rigor and informed by the best available evidence.

Many groups are using quality measure data to benchmark their performance against that of others. Despite this significant interest in benchmarking, we have relatively few valid and reliable measures of quality that are routinely measured and can be used to compare providers. Moreover, there is often uncertainty regarding the validity and reliability for a quality measure. Until the measures become robust, we must be cautious not to interpret them narrowly. We must allow the science to evolve. Another concern with the broad use of benchmarking is that although hospitals have limited resources for measuring quality, each stakeholder (purchasers such as the Leapfrog Group, regulators such as CMS, and accreditors such as JCAHO) has its own measures and its own definitions, increasing the compliance burden on hospitals and limiting providers' ability to use common measures. Recent collaborative efforts by these stakeholders and by the NQF to develop a common measure sheet should facilitate the development of common measures.

In addition to developing rigorous measures we need to learn how to report the results of these measures so they are most meaningful to consumers. Researchers should continue to explore how best to present quality data to consumers.

Despite these concerns the potential benefits are great. The performance feedback resulting from benchmarking can improve quality of care, and benchmarking will likely continue.

How Payors Use Benchmark Data

Given the magnitude of the quality and safety problem in health care, it is not surprising that many organizations, including health care purchasers, insurers, accreditors, and providers nationwide, are attempting to address this issue. One organization in particular, the Leapfrog Group, a consortium of over 150 Fortune 500 companies and large public employers, has focused on improving patient safety for its members' employees. For example, Leapfrog has created three hospital purchasing specifications for use by consumers and insurers that pay for employees' health care and also adopted the NQF safe practices (see Chapter Three) (Milstein and others, 2000).

The Leapfrog Group is growing daily and now addresses the needs of over thirty-five million employees from private and public employers such as Ford, Verizon, 3M, and the state of Massachusetts. Similar consortia, such as the Buyers Health Care Action Group and the Pacific Business Group on Health, are also Leapfrog Group members. Collectively, group members and their employees exercise significant purchasing power. In some market areas, employees of Leapfrog companies occupy a significant percentage of hospital beds. The consortium seeks to create a business case for quality by encouraging employees to use providers who have adopted transformational methods of performance improvement, a step providers are unlikely to take without a focused market reward.

The Leapfrog Group's three initial standards call for the following: (1) volume-based rules for specific neonatal care, (2) computerized physician order entry (CPOE) systems, and (3) higher levels of ICU physician staffing by intensive care physicians (*intensivists*). Implementing these standards in nonrural U.S. hospitals is expected to prevent 56,000 deaths a year, and most of this improvement is expected to result from improved ICU physician staffing (Provonost and others, 2002; Provonost and others, in press). To increase the number of hospitals meeting these standards, the Leapfrog Group implemented six regional *rollouts* in the past four years in which it partnered with regulators, insurers, and providers to support the implementation process.

The Leapfrog Group is using several methods to encourage members' employees to use hospitals that meet these standards. The group is working to increase public awareness of hospitals that meet the standards and is offering financial incentives and disincentives, such as an increased co-pay if an employee chooses a non-Leapfrog provider. Despite the magnitude of this endeavor, little is known about its impact on health care. Research is underway to measure the impact in the regions targeted for rollouts.

Even though the implementation and evaluation effort is ongoing, the Leapfrog standards have indeed become a benchmark, and failure to comply with these standards may increase an organization's liability exposure. Trial lawyers will likely interpret the Leapfrog standards as standards of care, further encouraging hospitals to implement these standards.

How Benchmark Data Become the Standard of Care

Benchmark data generally reflect a standard, a policy relating to a structural element of a hospital, or an empirical measure of quality. Performance on either an outside standard (such as a Leapfrog Group standard) or a quality outcome (that all patients with a myocardial infarction should receive beta-blockers, for example) can become a standard of care. When a standard is the benchmark, it generally represents the minimum performance that all hospitals should meet (for example, all hospitals should have an ethics committee). When an evidence-based process measure of quality of care is the benchmark, the standard of care is that all patients receive that process (such as receiving beta-blockers for myocardial infarction). Indeed, the standard of care is defined when the process measure is created. When an outcome measure (mortality, for example) is the benchmark, the outcomes of the top-performing organization often set that benchmark. Therefore the use of a quality measure rather than a standard as a benchmark may enhance quality by creating a maximum rather than minimum standard of care. Let's consider an example. One policy regarding infection control is that hospitals need an infection control program. The presence of an infection control program becomes the standard of care. Because most hospitals meet this, they would exceed the standard of care. However, if we use infection rates (such as rates of bloodstream infection) as the benchmark, the hospitals with the lowest infection rates create the standard of care; all those with higher rates may be perceived as failing to meet the standard.

One challenge in the use of benchmark data is to use them for learning rather than judging. Although using benchmark data for learning sounds like a straightforward concept, putting it into practice may require a shift in the culture of many health care organizations. Health care organizations have been judgmental of providers on a variety of issues, including resource utilization, performance, and economic credentialing. At the same time, health care providers have fought the idea of following one clinical approach or guideline, labeling such behavior *cookbook medicine*.

Benchmarking is supposed to go beyond judgmental appraisal. It does not set rigid parameters for measurement. Rather, when done appropriately, benchmarking supports a clinical framework that fosters quality care. Run charts, control charts, and statistical process controls (SPCs) are tools that can be used for this purpose. Measuring outcomes or performance over a period of time, providers can ascertain whether they have been within the benchmark criteria.

Providers have been hesitant to embrace benchmark concepts for a number of reasons. Distrust of the benchmark data and concern about flawed algorithms are key issues. If data are not risk adjusted or weighted correctly, a benchmark or algorithm may be set that is inaccurate and can lead to patient injury or to an incorrect decision to initiate a peer review process for some care providers. Payors relying on such information might terminate agreements or decide not to renew provider contracts. Provider concerns about benchmarking data must be addressed before there can be widespread acceptance of such information in revising guidelines for care. Gaining such support will require fulfilling a number of considerations, including the following:

- Agreement on a consistent methodology for setting benchmarks
- Agreement that clinical benchmarks be premised on a common set of factors, including quality, safety, and likelihood of successful outcome
- Development of benchmarks that are evidence based
- Definitions of what constitutes *evidence based*
- Consistent use of risk adjusting and weighting of data
- Recognition that a benchmark is a range of expected outcomes, leaving room for individual exceptions
- Provision for documenting the reason for an exception to the benchmark
- Use of exceptional cases and innovations to refresh the benchmark
- Education for those who use benchmark data, including demonstrated competency in using the information
- Establishment of a process for periodic evaluation and updating of evidence-based benchmarks

Health care facility executives and board members should understand that benchmarks can help them in meeting their obligations under federal and state law for the provision of quality assessment and performance improvement (QAPI) (68 *Fed. Reg.* 16, 3435–3455, Jan. 24, 2003). The results of benchmark data can guide future planning, budgeting, staffing, and operations. Good evidence-based outcomes can also be useful when contracting with payors. With public policy experts and lawmakers exploring revamping payment to reflect pay for performance, benchmark data take on added importance. Aligning economic incentives with patient safety will drive the change to evidence-based outcomes in the delivery of care.

How Consumers Use Benchmark Data

Quality data and benchmark information are important to many consumers. They want to know which hospital or provider has the best rating for performing certain types of surgeries or other specialized care. In selecting a nursing facility for a parent, they want to know which skilled facility has a positive rating. They look to the Centers for Medicare & Medicaid Services (2004) (which offer a service called Nursing Home Compare), several states (such as Virginia, 2004, and New York, 2004), and a number of national associations for such information. New private-public sector tools are also anticipated, including a national quality initiative (Centers for Medicare & Medicaid Services, 2004).

Just as providers need training for the interpretation of evidence-based data, the same is true of consumers. Information presented in a technical manner will do little to educate consumers. However a benchmark report card with a user-friendly format may encourage them to ask care providers for further information. Data about complications, length of stay, infection rates, and morbidity and mortality might lead to patients' rejecting one hospital or doctor and favoring another. Indeed, the communication of such information may become part of the consent process, to the extent that evidence-based clinical information shapes the discussion of the potential benefits and risks of a proposed treatment.

The possibility that benchmark data may provoke a shift in market share by changing the ways consumers make their choices may create a new incentive for improving patient safety. It is important for health care organizations and providers to make certain that benchmark data are understandable to all concerned. For example, they may wish to field-test the benchmark report card to evaluate the ability of consumers to interpret and use the data. This might be done in various sample population groups. Care providers then need to go one step further, learning from the data generated through examining evidence-based outcomes.

Conclusion: Using Benchmark Data to Achieve Patient Safety Compliance

The potential for using benchmark data to improve the quality of care is significant. Nevertheless, several prerequisites must be met before the improvements can be realized. First, each quality measure must be valid, reliable, and linked to meaningful improvements in safety. Second, a system must exist for sharing best practices among the sites participating in a benchmarking process. Third, providers must implement interventions and improve performance on each measure. They must avoid the common trap of allowing the collection of benchmark data to become an end in itself, with no link to improvement.

References

Centers for Medicare & Medicaid Services. "Nursing Home Compare." [http://www.medicare.gov/NHCompare/home.asp]. 2004.

Centers for Medicare & Medicaid Services. "The 'National Voluntary Hospital Reporting Initiative (NVHRI)' Will Now Be Known as 'Hospital Quality Alliance (HQA): Improving Care Through Information.'" [www.cms.hhs.gov/quality/hospital]. 2004.

Donabedian, A. "Evaluating Quality of Medical Care." *Milbank Quarterly*, 1966, *44*, 166–206.

Institute of Medicine. *Crossing the Quality Chasm: A New Health System for the 21st Century.* Washington, D.C.: National Academy Press, 2001.

Joint Commission on Accreditation of Healthcare Organizations. [http://www.jcaho.org]. 2004.

Leapfrog Group. "Purchasing Principles." [http://www.leapfroggroup.org/for_members/what_does_it_mean/purchasing_principals]. Jan. 2002.

Lohr, K. N., and Schroeder, S. A. "A Strategy for Quality Assurance in Medicare." *New England Journal of Medicine,* 1990, *322,* 1161–1171.

McGlynn, E. A. "Choosing and Evaluating Clinical Performance Measures." *Joint Commission Journal of Quality Improvement,* 1998, *24,* 470–479.

Milstein, A., and others. "Improving the Safety of Health Care: The Leapfrog Initiative." *Effective Clinical Practice,* 2000, *2*(6), 489–496.

New York State Department of Health. "New York State Physician Profile." [http://www.nydoctorprofile.com/about.jsp]. 2004.

Provonost, P. J., and others. "Physician Staffing Patterns and Clinical Outcomes in Critically Ill Patients: A Systematic Review," *The Journal of the American Medical Association,* 2002, *288*(17), 2151–2162.

Provonost, P. J., and others. "How Can Clinicians Measure Safety and Quality in Acute Care?" *Lancet,* 2004, *363*(9414), 1061–1067.

Provonost, P. J., and others. "Interventions to Reduce Mortality Among Patients Treated in Intensive Care Units." *Journal of Critical Care,* in press.

Rubin, H., Pronovost, P., and Diette, G. "From a Process of Care to a Measure: The Development and Testing of a Quality Indicator." *International Journal of Quality in Health Care,* 2001, *13*(6), 489–496.

Virginia Department of Health Professions. "Physician Information Project." [http://www.dhp.state.va.us]. 2004.

CHAPTER SEVEN

CREATION AND PRESERVATION OF REPORTS, DATA, AND DEVICE EVIDENCE IN MEDICAL ERROR SITUATIONS

Jane C. McConnell
Susan Durbin Kinter

Since the 1930s, health care and its delivery have undergone dramatic changes. With the introduction of private insurance funding for health care services, the advent of Medicare and Medicaid legislation, and the increase in federal funding for health research and the training of professionals, the entire health care industry gradually changed from a basically philanthropic one to a complex, business-oriented one. During this time, amazing diagnostic, therapeutic, and technological advances occurred enabling more people to be cured and live longer lives. With these medical advances, patients' expectations for recovery soared. The public's distrust of caregivers intensified, as expectations were not met and news of medical errors surfaced. This led to a general belief that health care providers cover up their mistakes. Publicity surrounding large settlements and jury awards rendered in medical malpractice cases has misguided the public into believing that treatment can always result in a good outcome and that if it doesn't someone did something wrong and should pay.

Despite these difficulties, health care institutions and providers continue to meet their obligation to improve care and reduce the potential for medical errors. The process involved in improving patient care and safety is complex. Any such process must include systems for identifying actual or potential risk areas and medical error situations and evaluating the success of any action plans designed to respond to the risk areas identified.

One of the most basic means of identifying risk areas in the health care system is the *incident report*. Historically, this has been the main document for reporting adverse events and departures from the standard of care. Unfortunately, the reporting system in the past has been associated with punitive actions on the part of management. In addition the information generated was often inaccurate, and because an individual was always to blame, no system issues were addressed. Therefore many events went unreported (Brennan and others, 1991, p. 370). Today there has been significant change in the process. The barriers to reporting have been reduced, encouraging more frequent reporting. A culture of blame-free reporting associated with accountability, compassion, and concern must now be introduced.

The incident report may be used in a plethora of ways to reduce risk areas and improve patient care. If the information gathered from incident reports is maintained in a data system, that information can be analyzed and problem areas and trends can be identified. Data specific to patient care units can be generated and discussed with the individuals managing the units. Patient safety initiatives formulated to address specific problems identified in an institution can be used to prevent future injury. In addition data can be analyzed to determine the effectiveness of action plans already in place. The data gathered through incident reporting can be incorporated in quality and risk reports that can be shared with individuals and committees whose purpose is to promote safe, quality care. The incident report can be the catalyst for an investigation of an event that has the potential for litigation. Things learned from the incident report can be used in the education of staff with the hope of preventing future adverse events or medical errors.

Incident reports may be an invaluable tool, but in order to use them successfully the organization must have an incident reporting process in place. This process should address training staff in how to use the incident report, communicating about the adverse-event or medical error situation recorded in the incident report, investigating the adverse event, if appropriate, and assessing the potential for litigation associated with the adverse event. The incident reporting process must also have in place mechanisms for keeping the information learned and data collected confidential.

Incident Reporting Process Overview

The incident reporting process begins with identifying the types of events the institution wishes to capture through the incident report. Does the institution wish to capture adverse events, medication errors, or near-miss situations? The term *adverse event* may have a variety of meanings, ranging from care that results in a minor injury to a patient (for example, a patient falls while on fall precautions but suffers no injury) to a devastating outcome for a patient. A near miss occurs when there is a deviation from the standard of care (for example, a nurse administers a wrong medication to a patient) but there is no injury to the patient.

A serious adverse event, when the patient's outcome is significantly worse than anticipated, can occur in the presence or absence of negligence (that is, whether the standard of care was not or was adhered to). The severity of the event often dictates what action will be taken. However serious the event, the first action to be taken is to ensure that the patient is receiving the appropriate treatment. Once the patient's immediate needs have been addressed, the process of managing the adverse event should begin.

The initial step in managing an adverse event is to report it to the appropriate individuals. Every institution should have a policy or practice in place outlining how and to whom an adverse event should be reported. Events can be reported through incident reports. In addition, events can be called in to the appropriate personnel. Some institutions have implemented on-line reporting. Whatever mechanism is used to report events, institutions must train their personnel on the importance of reporting these events. Such training should include identification of the adverse events the institution wishes to capture. For example, if the institution wishes to capture near-miss events, that should be explicitly articulated. Because there is no patient injury associated with a near-miss event, this type of event is not regularly reported despite the opportunity it gives the organization to put a corrective action plan in place before an actual patient injury occurs.

Individuals should be instructed in how to write an incident report. Incident reports should contain a brief objective recitation of the event. The information contained in the incident report should be factual, objective, and not unlike what is written in the patient's chart. In addition, the incident report should contain only those facts known at the time. There should be no speculation about how the incident occurred or what injury possibly resulted. Incident reports should not contain blameful, accusatory, or finger-pointing language. The incident report should never be kept as part of the medical record. Printing the incident report on colored paper is helpful in keeping the incident report separate from the medical record as it can then easily be identified. Once an incident report is completed, the institution should have in place a process detailing where the report goes. Often the incident report will go first to the nurse manager or supervisor of the unit where the incident occurred. This enables the nurse manager to learn of the adverse event and then take immediate action in response. From there the incident report may be forwarded to the quality management or risk management department, depending on the institution's procedures.

Whatever the process the incident report should be completed and forwarded to the appropriate individuals in a timely fashion. Once received by the quality management or, usually, risk management department, the incident report will be reviewed, and if appropriate, an investigation of the incident will occur. The investigation may range from relatively simple (a review of the medical record) to complex (with interviews of involved staff and an expert review). Specific directions for conducting an investigation are discussed later in this chapter.

After an investigation is completed, an evaluation of the adverse incident must occur. Ideally, during the evaluation the incident will be given a severity code that can be used in data retrieval and reporting. For instance, if the institution wishes to monitor poor patient outcomes regardless of standard of care or policy and procedure violations, the focus of the severity code can be the type of injury a patient suffered. If the institution wishes to capture near-miss events in its data system, the severity code can reflect that purpose. For instance, a 1 might represent no or unknown criticisms of care, with no injury; 2 might represent no criticisms of care, with injury; 3 might represent criticisms of care, with no injury; and 4 might represent criticisms of care, with an injury. In this scenario, a 3 would be used to capture a near-miss situation and a 4 to capture an incident having a potential for litigation.

The evaluation should analyze whether the incident requires any corrective action, and if so, who should be engaged to formulate the corrective action plan and be accountable for its completion. If individuals who have the power to create change are not part of this process, change is unlikely to occur. Therefore it is important to involve individuals both committed to the process and empowered to take the necessary action. The evaluation should also determine whether the incident is significant enough to justify attaching some monetary value to it (this practice is commonly referred to as placing a *reserve* on it). Some institutions may wish to place a reserve on an incident having a potential for litigation (for example, one that may result in a claim or lawsuit), whereas other institutions may refrain from this practice. This decision may be made either within the institution if it is self-insured or outside the institution if it is commercially insured or outsources its claims management.

Proactive Steps to Identify Risk Areas

As we stated earlier, the incident report is the primary tool used by health care institutions to identify risk areas in the institution. In addition to analyzing the data learned from incident reports, institutions can proactively examine information from several other sources to identify risk areas. Sources other than the incident report that are internal to the institution and available to identify actual or potential risk areas include morbidity and mortality conferences, quality management meetings, quality of care or sentinel event reviews, and institutional committee meetings. Risk managers and quality care professionals should attend such meetings to gather information on actual medical errors and near misses that they might otherwise not have been made aware of. In addition meetings addressing pharmacy issues can provide information about such things as drug recalls, adverse drug reactions, and medical errors or delays, if such information is not routinely reported to the risk management or quality department. Lastly, the medical records department of the institution should be instructed to forward to the department of risk management all medical record requests received from well-known plaintiff law firms in the area. Although many of these medical record requests may not relate to potential litigation against the institution, this is a worthwhile endeavor because there will be situations in which an incident report was not completed on a patient who had an adverse event, and if the risk management department receives notice of a medical record request, the incident can be investigated prior to notification of a lawsuit.

Several external sources are also available to identify actual or potential risk areas and medical error situations. When the institution is insured through a commercial insurer, insurance professionals (carriers, brokers, and consultants) can carry out a review of the institution to identify potential risk areas. The Joint Commission on Accreditation of Healthcare Organizations (hereinafter Joint Commission or JCAHO) publishes *Sentinel Event Alerts*. A *sentinel event* is "an unexpected occurrence involving death or serious physical or psychological injury, or the risk thereof" (JCAHO, 2002). *Sentinel Event Alerts* can inform an institution of risk areas identified through the experience of other institutions. Published for organizations accredited by the Joint Commission, these alerts identify specific sentinel events and describe their common underlying causes in addition to suggesting steps to prevent such occurrences in the future. Accordingly, institutions receiving these alerts have the opportunity to correct a potential patient safety concern before any patient is injured. Other organizations, such as the American Society for Healthcare Risk Management (ASHRM, 2004), also have publications discussing risk areas and medical errors experienced by member institutions.

Proactive Steps to Manage an Adverse Event

When an adverse event or medical error occurs, specific proactive steps need to be taken both on the institutional and the risk management levels. The following sections address these steps.

Reporting the Event

On the institutional level the institution should have a policy or guideline in place giving direction to institution personnel about the steps to be taken when an adverse event or medical error occurs. This policy should identify the people and functions that should be notified (for example, representatives of the hospital administration, risk management, and media relations). The institution should also have a policy in place directing that the incident or event be reported to the department of risk management within twenty-four hours. If an adverse event occurs after business hours, the policy should direct the provider to call the administrator on call or an individual acting in that capacity. Lastly, the institution should have a policy or guideline in place addressing disclosure of an unexpected outcome. JCAHO and ASHRM have written materials addressing this policy. The policy should identify who will be responsible for the disclosure, when the disclosure will take place, and what information will be disclosed. (For additional information about disclosure see Chapter Nine.)

Investigating the Event

Once the incident is reported, an initial determination must be made about whether the incident needs to be investigated. If there is a significant injury to the patient, some form of investigation is probably warranted. If, however, the event is a relatively minor one, a patient fell and did not harm himself, for example, an investigation may not be warranted. Whether an investigation needs to occur immediately will depend on the facts of the event. If the event involves a clear deviation from the standard of care that resulted in a patient death or serious injury, or if it involves a probable equipment malfunction that resulted in serious patient harm or death, an immediate investigation is warranted.

When an adverse event or medical error occurs, there are key strategies to employ for information gathering. The investigator should obtain and review the medical record, especially such items as X-ray films, fetal monitoring tracings, or any other pertinent part of the record. He or she should review the medical record in order to ensure that it is complete. If the proper entries have not been made, staff who have failed to make a necessary entry in the record should be directed to make their notation in the chart. Late-entry notes should be made in a timely fashion, within forty-eight hours of the event. These notes should be identified as late-entry notes and be factual and objective in their content. They should not contain information that could be characterized as defensive or self-serving. Whether or not to write a late-entry note may be a question. Should an adverse event later result in litigation, a late-entry note rarely assists a defendant health care provider in that litigation. Plaintiff's lawyers and jurors often look on late-entry notes suspiciously. Accordingly, in writing a late-entry note one should seriously consider the purpose of the note and what benefit, if any, such a note would be in the ongoing treatment of the patient. Involved staff may need assistance in writing a note in the record about the adverse event or medical error.

If the investigation reveals that the incident is likely to result in agitation or litigation, sequester all parts of the medical record, including X-ray films, fetal monitoring strips, and the like. Include all "loose filing" and any parts of the medical record that have not made it to the chart. This should ensure that the records will not be misplaced should litigation later arise. Make certain that a formal process for sequestration is in place; do not simply have someone put the record "in a safe place," as the safe place may be forgotten as time goes by. Instruct the medical records department to notify risk management should the patient or an attorney request the sequestered record. The request for sequestration should not be kept as part of the medical record.

The importance of having a formal process in place for sequestration of medical records and other material significant to an investigation is demonstrated by the case of *Timothy Laubach et al.* v. *Franklin Square Hospital* (1989). In *Laubach* a hospital was found in violation of a state statute governing the disclosure of medical records when the hospital could not locate, and therefore could not produce, fetal monitoring strips in a timely fashion. Although the hospital produced the medical record, it did not produce the fetal monitoring strips for seventy-eight days. Finding that the hospital violated the state statute, a jury awarded the plaintiffs $1 million in compensatory and punitive damages. This award was upheld on appeal. In addition to a possible statutory violation claim (as was brought in *Laubach*), hospitals are at risk of a spoliation of evidence claim if they cannot locate pieces of the medical record during litigation. The impact of a spoliation claim is often determined by state statute or case law and varies among states, but it can also certainly act to prejudice a jury against a defendant.

Once the medical record has been reviewed, the involved staff should be interviewed. These interviews may be conducted in-house by risk management or may be outsourced. In determining how these interviews will be conducted, take into consideration whether they will be protected. State law should give guidance on whether interviews of staff members conducted as part of a quality review or risk management investigation will be protected. The quality of the interviews will likely depend not only on the experience of the interviewer but also on the level of trust developed between the health care providers and the department of risk management. In order to promote a trusting relationship, involved staff members should be informed that these interviews are confidential and that the source of any information learned will not be revealed. Instruct the involved staff not to discuss the event among themselves informally. They should also be instructed that if anyone outside the institution and the investigation should contact them, they are not to discuss the incident. In addition, instruct the staff not to keep personal notes memorializing the event, as commonly such notes are not protected. Lastly, instruct the staff that if they leave the institution they are to notify the department of risk management of a forwarding address should they need to be contacted in the future.

If the event involves a medical device, additional action is required. The device should be removed from service and sequestered. The institution's biomedical engineering department should be notified. Oftentimes when a manufacturer is advised of a problem with one of its devices, it will ask that the device be returned to it. Do not return the device to the manufacturer or allow the manufacturer to test, clean, or alter the device unless you are advised to do so by your institution's insurance carrier or defense attorney or until you have obtained advice from an independent biomedical expert. Should the malfunctioning of the device result in litigation, often the manufacturer's interest is adverse to that of the institution. Consider whether consulting with an outside expert such as ECRI would be appropriate. ECRI, formerly known as the Emergency Care Research Institute, is an independent, nonprofit health services agency whose mission is to improve the safety, quality, and cost effectiveness of health care. Although engaging an independent expert is an added expense, he or she can often tell you whether the device malfunctioned (as opposed to user error) and whether other institutions have had similar problems with this or similar medical equipment or devices. Consider whether it is necessary to report the event to the Food and Drug Administration (FDA) pursuant to the Safe Medical Devices Act (discussed later in this chapter). Obtain copies of and sequester any and all maintenance records and rental or purchase agreements related to the device. Lastly, determine whether any medical device alerts were issued by the manufacturer, the distributor, or the FDA and who in your institution is responsible for acting on such alerts.

Once the medical record has been reviewed and the involved health care personnel have been interviewed, determine whether an expert review is warranted. If there is any question whether the standard of care was breached, obtain an expert review. Expert reviews may also be helpful in determining whether the action or omission by the health care provider resulted in any injury to the patient. Again, it must be stressed that these expert reviews are to be confidential, and the expert reviewer is not to discuss the case with any colleague inside or outside the institution.

Communicating About the Event

Information about the event will need to be communicated to various organizations and individuals at some point during the investigation or at its completion. The extent and content of the communication will depend on the severity of the event. Determine who should be informed of the event. If the institution is commercially insured and if the event is a serious one, the event should be reported to the primary and excess insurance carriers as soon as possible. If the event has resulted in the death of a patient, an immediate assessment of the need to communicate the event to the medical examiner or coroner must be made; individual state statutes may give guidance on the types of death that must be reported. Your institution's policies may address this as well.

An early assessment should be made to identify which, if any, hospital administrators, senior management, and media relations personnel need to be informed of the event. If it is necessary to notify media relations, determine whether a spokesperson should be identified. If a spokesperson is selected, formulate a response to both internal and external inquiries. Again, if the institution is commercially insured, the insurance carrier should be kept informed of and involved in these decisions. Assess whether abating insurance or patient bills is appropriate, and if so, notify the individual responsible for this task. Lastly, assess the need to involve law enforcement. The appropriate law enforcement officials should be notified when the incident involves known or suspected criminal activity, for example, in cases of complaints of assault of a patient by another patient or institution employee.

Usually, an evaluation of the need to notify the patient or family about the adverse event must occur early in the process. Although disclosure of adverse events and outcomes is discussed in more detail in Chapter Nine, it is appropriate to briefly address communicating adverse events to patients and families here. Unfortunately, in the heat of the moment, health care providers often make errors that compromise a later investigation of the event. In an effort to defuse the anxious situation when a patient or patient's family is asking what happened, often several different health care providers will relay to a patient or family member their understanding of the way an event occurred. When these health care providers were not actually present at the time the event occurred and thus may not have knowledge of all the pertinent facts, the patient or family may receive several differing accounts of how the event occurred. This may not only confuse the family or the patient but may also raise questions in the patient's or a family member's mind about the veracity of the information told to them. For this reason it is recommended that when an adverse event occurs, one person be designated as responsible for communicating information to the patient or family. This individual should disclose to the patient or his or her family only information known at the time. As with the incident report, this disclosure should not speculate as to how the incident occurred or whether there is any causative connection between the incident and any injury the patient may have sustained. Frequently, patients or their families are misinformed about events and their consequences by well-intentioned health care providers who think they are aiding the family when in reality they are speculating about both how the event occurred and its effect. Such misinformation can have a devastating impact on the defense of any litigation that may arise from the incident.

Strategies for Preserving Evidence

Although the majority of incidents reported do not result in litigation, today's society is a litigious one where most if not all incidents have the potential for litigation. Accordingly, institutions must have in place a system for preserving what may later become evidence in a malpractice lawsuit: medical records, X-rays, fetal monitoring tracings, other patient care records, and all medical devices. Determine what is to be put in writing and how much should be included in various reports. Staff interviews and expert reviews should be put in writing so that the information is available in the future. Keep in mind, however, that whether such material is protected is dependent on state law and how the information is managed. Remember, no matter what protections are available to keep material confidential, a judge, at his or her discretion, can order the material turned over in litigation. Keep this thought in mind whenever anything is written down. In addition, if the information gathered as a result of a risk management investigation is shared, either through a written report or verbally, individuals must be instructed that they cannot share that information either intentionally or inadvertently (for example, by leaving a copy of a risk management report in an open area after a quality meeting has taken place); if they do, any privilege that might have attached to the material will be considered waived.

Likewise, be cautious about who reviews these materials. Do not unwittingly waive any privilege that might have attached to certain material by allowing someone outside the process to see it, as that triggers the privilege to review these materials. For instance, allowing a staff member who has been interviewed to review her interview to refresh her recollection may waive the privilege that otherwise would have deemed that interview confidential.

Once the information is obtained, determine who should maintain that information. Should the information be kept at the institution? If so, determine how long the information should be kept on site, and place it in a fireproof, waterproof, locked storage file. If the information is going to be kept off site because the investigation has been outsourced to a defense firm, insurance company, or other contractual agency, determine what information the risk management or quality department should review and how that information should be stored. If the department of risk management stores any investigation files off site, at a storage facility for example, have a process in place for keeping track of where the file has gone and when. Should litigation later arise, this investigation file will be most helpful in piecing together how the event occurred. If it is the practice to destroy investigation files or any reports generated from risk management data after a certain amount of time, make certain the institution has a policy in place delineating when these files will be destroyed and under what conditions.

When the incident involves a medical device, additional action must be taken, as described earlier: sequester the device and any and all maintenance records and rental or purchase agreements immediately; determine whether any medical device alerts were issued by the manufacturer, the distributor, or the FDA; and identify who is responsible for acting on such alerts.

Strategies for Keeping Information Confidential

Know the strategies available to your institution for keeping information confidential. State law and federal law will mandate what can be considered confidential. Determine whether your state has legislation making certain processes and materials confidential. Most states have such legislation, and these laws will define the materials and processes that are protected. For example, state legislation may protect peer review committees,[1] quality assurance committees,[2] quality management programs,[3] quality review programs,[4] risk management proceedings,[5] and hospital medical staff committee proceedings.[6] One must look at the language of the relevant statute to determine exactly what is protected.

In order to preserve protections created by statute, it is helpful to label documents and relevant policies and procedures with language similar to that of the statute. For example, legislation enacted in New Hampshire (*N.H. Rev. Stat. Ann.* § 151:13-a [II], 2003) states that records of a hospital committee organized to evaluate matters relating to the care and treatment of patients and testimony of individuals appearing before or participating in a quality assurance committee is "confidential," "privileged," and shall be inadmissible in any judicial or administrative process. Because the statute specifically refers to a quality assurance committee, all incident reports compiled for such groups and other reports of such groups should be labeled, "confidential, privileged for the purpose of quality assurance."

Also look to the statute to determine the scope of any protection. For instance, some statutes may exclude from protection any records or materials that have not been generated as part of the protected process and are otherwise available (as is the case, for example, in Maryland; see, *Md. Code Ann., Health Occ.* § 14-501[e], 2004). Medical records are an example of excluded materials. Because the medical record of a patient is generated outside the peer review process, protected status would not attach to a medical record simply because it is used in a risk management investigation. That is why incident reports should never be kept as part of the original medical record. Simply labeling them "confidential" or "privileged" or as part of a quality assurance program is not likely to result in their being deemed confidential.

Materials created specifically for quality assurance or risk management programs, if identified in terms mirroring a state statute offering such materials protection, will most likely be deemed protected if they are requested by someone outside the quality assurance or risk management process. Many documents are created during the course of caring for a patient that might not always be made a part of the medical record yet are not created specifically for a peer review, risk management, or quality of care process. Whether protected status will attach to these documents must be analyzed on a case-by-case basis. A patient experiences cardiac arrest, for example. After a code has been called and resuscitation has been unsuccessful, one of the staff who responded to the code prints the memory from the cardiac monitor to better understand what happened with the patient. An investigation reveals that the patient's alarm was activated for ten minutes before any health care provider responded. This information was learned only through reviewing the memory from the cardiac monitor. The patient's family, unaware that the monitor was not responded to in a timely fashion, but angry over their loved one's death, sues the institution. During the course of the litigation "all medical records, printouts, and other documents related to the care of the patient" are requested. The relevant state statute protects all quality assurance and peer review materials. In the attempt to determine whether the monitor printout would fall within the protected category, the staff are interviewed. They report that they routinely print out a monitor's history after a code is called because it is helpful in documenting the patient's course; they do not print it out strictly for quality assurance purposes. In this example the monitor history would likely have to be produced despite the state statute governing quality assurance and peer review activities. If, however, during an investigation it is learned that the cardiac monitor printout is not routinely obtained and was obtained in this case solely to evaluate the health care provider's response to a monitor alarm, the protection may attach.

Again, even when documents are deemed confidential by a state statute, that privilege can be waived inadvertently if the documents or interviews are sent to individuals outside the process that affords them protection. For instance, a nurse, angry that a physician failed to respond to her multiple pages when her patient's condition deteriorated, writes an incident report. Instead of following the procedure of sending the incident report directly to risk management, she makes several copies and forwards a copy of the incident report to the chairperson of the physician's department and the chief executive officer of the institution. Although these individuals obviously have an interest in institutional quality issues, they have no direct quality assurance or risk management duties. By sending the chairperson and the CEO a copy of the incident report, the nurse has potentially waived the privilege that otherwise might have attached to that document.

In addition, as mentioned previously, even when a state statute deems certain materials confidential, a judge may still order disclosure. In the case of *Livotte* v. *New York City Health and Hospitals Corporation* (1989), a U.S. District Court ordered that incident reports prepared by five New York hospitals be produced, despite a state statute declaring such reports privileged. The court based its finding on its previous finding that disclosure was not likely to cause any discernable injury to the state policy of encouraging full reporting of such incidents (*Livotte*, 1989, p. 2) and that there was an inadequate showing to overcome the rebuttable presumption in a federal case that relevant documents that are not subject to a federally recognized privilege are discoverable, not withstanding the existence of a state law privilege (Livotte, 1989, p. 3). Thus, despite a clear statute affording protection to the incident reports, a judge, applying a different standard, deemed the privilege inapplicable in a specific circumstance.

In states affording no protections to quality review committees, peer review committees, and the like, other avenues must be considered to protect the information from discovery during litigation. Treating serious incidents as if they will result in litigation may be one avenue to protection. Sending incident reports to outside counsel or to a medical malpractice insurer and having outside counsel or the insurer investigate the incident and interview involved providers may attach a protection to these materials. Although potentially costly, such action may enable the institution to conduct a full investigation and learn facts surrounding the event without compromising its ability to defend itself should litigation later arise.

Many states including Connecticut have mandatory reporting requirements. A Connecticut statute provides a limited protection to health care institutions that identify and report medical errors to the public health commissioner. The law prevents information collected from subpoena, discovery, or introduction into evidence in any judicial or administrative proceeding. Some exceptions are built into the law. The Connecticut approach may reflect a good compromise between evidentiary protection and gathering medical error information to be used in improving patient safety.

Reporting Incidents, Adverse Events, and Medical Errors

Both the federal government and many state governments have passed legislation to codify their interest in acquiring better information about events that affect patient safety. The following sections offer an introduction to this legislation.

State Reporting

In 1999, the Institute of Medicine issued a report (Kohn, Corrigan, and Donaldson, 2000) calling national attention to the relationship between medical errors in hospitals and hospital deaths. The report proclaimed that medical errors are a leading cause of death in the United States. Since that report was published, many states have enacted legislation addressing medical errors, presumably with the goal of promoting greater patient safety in the delivery of health care and the reduction of such errors. As of September 2001, over half of the states (twenty-six) require some type of reporting. Of these twenty-six, twenty-four have enacted mandatory reporting requirements,[7] and two have voluntary reporting legislation.[8] The remaining twenty-four states and the District of Columbia have no reporting requirements.

As has been noted, the type (mandatory or voluntary) of reporting required by individual states varies, as does the need to report. What must be reported is also variable. Vague terms such as "incident,"[9] "accident" or "unusual occurrence,"[10] "potential injury,"[11] and "quality of care problems,"[12] are used in some state statutes. Other state statutes are more specific, using such terms as "medical error,"[13] "adverse event,"[14] "medication error,"[15] and "death."[16] Some state statutes are very explicit in their reporting requirements. For instance, Rhode Island's statute specifically defines what must be reported: "any incident causing or involving brain injury, unexpected patient death, mental impairment, paraplegia, quadriplegia, paralysis, loss of use of limb or organ, birth injury, surgery on the wrong patient, impairment of sight or hearing, or subjecting a patient to a procedure that was not ordered or intended by the physician" (1956 *R.I. Gen. Laws* § 23-17-40, 2003). The same section of the Rhode Island statute also requires that these incidents be reported within seventy-two hours to the Department of Health and Human Services. The statute does afford protection to the proceedings and records generated as a result of peer review activities. Such materials are protected from discovery in a medical malpractice action and should be inadmissible in a medical malpractice trial.

The person or organization designated to receive reported information also varies from state to state. Many state statutes require that the required disclosure be made to the state health department or a hybrid thereof.[17] Other states require merely that the information be reported to a source internal to the institution gathering the information.[18] Whatever the requirement, it is essential that institutions have in place a process to ensure compliance with any statute or regulation placed upon them at the state level.

Federal Reporting

In addition to reporting adverse events and medical errors at the state level as required, health care institutions must comply with reporting requirements based on federal law and with requests for voluntary reports at the national level.

Reporting Pursuant to the Safe Medical Devices Act. The Safe Medical Devices Act (SMDA) was promulgated in 1990 and increased the Food and Drug Administration's regulatory authority over the medical device industry. The Act was amended in 1992 with a uniform definition for *serious injury* and *serious illness* as these terms relate to manufacturer and user facility reporting.

The SMDA requires hospitals, nursing homes, outpatient treatment centers, and ambulatory surgery facilities to report incidents in which it is believed that a device may have caused or contributed to the death of a patient or a serious patient injury. A *serious illness* or *serious injury* is defined by the Act as an "illness or injury that is life threatening or that either results in permanent impairment of bodily function or permanent damage to a bodily structure or necessitates immediate medical or surgical intervention to avoid permanent impairment of a bodily function or permanent damage to a bodily structure." The term *medical device* "includes but is not limited to ventilators, monitors, dialyzers, and any other electronic equipment, implants, thermometers, patient restraints, syringes, catheters, in vitro diagnostic test kits and reagents, disposables, components, parts, accessories and related software." In cases involving the death of a patient, the institution must report the death within ten days to the manufacturer *and* the FDA. In cases where the patient is injured or becomes seriously ill but does not die, a report must be filed within ten working days with the manufacturer *or* with the FDA if the manufacturer is unknown.

The SMDA also requires that implantable devices be tracked by the institution. Every trackable device must be listed in a patient's medical record, in the hospital's purchasing or accounting system, and in the manufacturer's records. Hospitals must inform manufacturers of patients' names, identity of devices, lot and serial numbers, and implantation dates.

In order to comply with the Safe Medical Devices Act, institutions must have in place a policy or procedure to ensure the proper follow-up and investigation of any incident related to the failure or suspected failure of a medical device. The procedure should identify the department responsible for reporting medical device adverse events under the SMDA. It may be the risk management department or the biomedical engineering department. The institution must also make a summary report of all reports previously filed every six months (January 1 and July 1). The institution may make a report pursuant to the SMDA either in writing (the FDA has forms for this purpose) or on line.

Although the Safe Medical Devices Act promises the FDA's understanding and cooperation in keeping reported data confidential, the Act has many exceptions under which information can be released to various parties. In addition, if plaintiffs know what to ask for, they could request a copy of the institution's semiannual report to the FDA. Whether this is protected may depend on who is responsible for maintaining these reports. If, for example, an institution's biomedical engineering department is responsible for maintaining these reports, the reports may not be protected. If the reports are made pursuant to a process protected by state law, for example, as part of the institution's risk management or quality assurance plan, a privilege may attach to them.

When medical device failure does not result in serious injury, illness, or death, the institution may still report the failure voluntarily. When it is believed that a medical device has failed, it would be prudent to report that failure under any circumstance. Because the SMDA was designed to ensure the safety and effectiveness of medical devices through the monitoring of reports, patient safety can be further advanced by institutions' reporting efforts. In addition, if a lawsuit later arises out of the failure of a medical device, the fact that a report was filed under the SMDA might indicate that the institution felt that any alleged patient injury was related to device failure as opposed to user error. Plaintiffs can verify that an event report was submitted to the Food and Drug Administration by querying the FDA database under the Freedom of Information Act. If the event was reported, the FDA will have that report; if it was not reported and it was a serious event, then the institution becomes vulnerable in that it has not complied with the SMDA.

Reporting Pursuant to MedWatch. In addition to medical devices, the FDA also has responsibility for ensuring the safety and efficiency of all related marketed medical products, including prescription and over-the-counter drugs, biologics (for example, blood products), medical and radiation-emitting devices, and special nutritional products (for example, medical foods, dietary supplements, and infant formulas). MedWatch is the FDA's safety information and adverse-event reporting program that permits health care professionals and consumers to report serious problems that they believe are associated with the drugs and medical devices they prescribe, dispense, or use.

There are both voluntary and mandatory reporting requirements under MedWatch. Institutions are required to report suspected medical device–related deaths to both the FDA and the manufacturer, and serious injuries to the manufacturer or to the FDA, if the manufacturer is unknown. Suspected medical device–related deaths and serious injuries (if the manufacturer is unknown) can be reported to the FDA using MedWatch 3500, a mandatory reporting form. If an institution suspects a serious adverse event is associated with a drug, it can voluntarily report that event to the FDA using the MedWatch 3500 form. The institution's name and the name of anyone associated with the event are not identified on the MedWatch forms. To that extent the information is confidential.

A report to MedWatch is required only when one or more of the following occurs: (1) *an adverse reaction:* if a patient has an adverse reaction to a medical product and the reaction is a suspected cause of the patient's death, reporting is required; (2) *a life-threatening hazard:* if the patient was at risk of dying at the time of the adverse reaction or if it is suspected that continued use of the product would cause death, reporting is required (an example would be pacemaker breakdown or failure of an intravenous pump that could have caused excessive drug dosing); (3) *hospitalization:* if a patient is admitted to a hospital or has a prolonged hospital stay because of a serious adverse reaction, reporting is required; (4) *disability:* if a patient has an adverse reaction causing significant or permanent change in his or her body function, physical activities, or quality of life, reporting is required; (5) *birth defects, miscarriage, stillbirth, or birth with disease:* if exposure to a medical product before conception or during pregnancy is suspected of causing an adverse outcome in the child, reporting is required (an example would be malformation in a child caused by the acne drug Accutane); or (6) *intervention required to avoid permanent damage:* if use of a medical product required medical or surgical treatment to prevent impairment, reporting is necessary (examples would be burns from radiation equipment and a break in a screw supporting a bone fracture). The Food and Drug Administration emphasizes that it is not necessary to prove that a medical product caused an adverse reaction; suspected association is sufficient to trigger a report.

The identity of patients and other persons making MedWatch reports is kept confidential. The FDA does have regulations in place to preserve privacy. To report, log on to the FDA Web site (http://www.fda.gov/medwatch.com) and follow the instructions for submitting a report electronically. A report can also be mailed on a postage-paid MedWatch form that includes the address (obtain forms from MedWatch at 800-332-1088). You can also download the software for printing out the form (http://www.fda.gov/medwatch.com) or request a copy of the software on disk (301-443-0117). Completed forms may also be faxed to MedWatch (800-332-0178).

Voluntary Reporting

In addition to meeting mandatory state and federal reporting requirements, institutions may make voluntary reports. Agencies seeking voluntary institutional reporting include MEDMARX and the Joint Commission on Accreditation of Healthcare Organizations.

MEDMARX (http://www.medmarx.com) is a reporting system designed to augment, not replace, MedWatch. It is an Internet-accessible database that hospitals may use to report and track drug errors anonymously. MEDMARX allows hospitals to internally monitor the progress of their error prevention strategies, to share their successes with others, and to learn about the problems and solutions experienced by other institutions. The program promotes total anonymity. Confidentiality is achieved through assigning each subscriber a random, system-generated, confidential identification number that the subscriber then uses to access the system and transact within it. No third parties have access to MEDMARX data. Reporting is voluntary; however, there is a subscriber cost associated with its use.

The Joint Commission on Accreditation of Healthcare Organizations holds itself out as the nation's predominant standard-setting and accrediting body in health care. If an institution is accredited by JCAHO, then that institution must comply with the JCAHO sentinel event policy that requires institutions to conduct an intensive assessment of all serious adverse events. A sentinel event, as mentioned earlier, is defined by JCAHO as "an unexpected occurrence involving death or serious physical or psychological injury, or the risk thereof." The sentinel event policy also encourages, but does not mandate, institutions to report all sentinel events, along with the institution's root cause analysis and related preventive actions. Thus these reports are strictly voluntary.

Whether the self-critical analysis required under JCAHO's sentinel event policy is protected or not often will depend on any state protections that may attach to risk management or peer review activities or the like. There is not much case law discussing protections of the self-critical analysis. One New Jersey court, in an unpublished opinion, did address this issue in determining whether information a hospital obtained during its self-critical analysis of a patient death was discoverable in litigation surrounding the death (*Frank Reyes et al. v. Meadowlands Hospital Medical Center*, 2001). The court first looked to whether any statutory protections attached to the self-critical analysis process and found that although the Joint Commission had sought congressional recognition of a privilege in the form of legislation, no such legislation was forthcoming. The court next reviewed whether a privilege attached at the state level and found that no state statute acted to make such information protected from discovery. The court then looked to whether case law supported making such information confidential. Despite a previous opinion issued by the New Jersey Superior Court holding that discovery of similar material would impede a hospital's ability to candidly review the quality of care it rendered, the court held that self-analysis material should be disclosed.

Conclusion

Much legislation has been proposed on the federal level to further ensure patient safety. This legislation would address primarily medical error reporting and data protection. Risk managers must be on the alert for new legislation that may place additional reporting requirements on their institutions.

There is no question that patient safety is a priority on both the state and federal level. To comply with the many reporting requirements placed on them as a result of patient safety initiatives, health care institutions must have systems in place to ensure that adverse patient events (however each institution wishes to define them—and it is recommended that any definition conform to reporting requirements) are identified. Institutions are being called on not only to identify adverse patient events but also to have systems in place to investigate each event and correct any system flaw that may have contributed to that event. Although on their face such requirements would appear to be beneficial, unless such activity carries with it protections shielding institutions from having to disclose materials generated during these investigations, an institution's ability to defend itself in any subsequent litigation will be greatly compromised. A balance must be reached between an institution's ability to set in place processes promoting patient safety and the institution's need to protect information gathered in such processes. Many states offer protections to an institution's internal activities to promote safe, quality care. Institutions must look to any protections afforded them and incorporate those protections in their patient safety initiatives.

Notes

1. See *Haw. Rev. Stat. Ann.* § 671D (2003); *Iowa Code* § 147.135 (2004).
2. See *Haw. Rev. Stat. Ann.* § 663-1.7 (2003).
3. See *Colo. Rev. Stat. Ann.* § 25-3-209 (2004).
4. See *Del. Code Ann.* § 9707 (2003).
5. See *Fla. Stat. Ann.* § 395.0197 (2004).
6. See *Idaho Code* § 39-1392 (2003).
7. States having mandatory reporting requirements include Arizona, *Ariz. Rev. Stat.* R9-20-111; Arkansas, *Ark. Code Ann.* §§ 20-7-302–305 (1987–2003); California Senate Bill (CA SB) 1875 (2000); Colorado, *Colo. Rev. Stat.* § 25-1-124 (2004); Connecticut, General Stat. § 19a-127n, as amended by Pub Act 04-164 (2004); Florida, *Fla. Admin. Code Ann.* r. 59a-10.0055 (2004); Georgia, *Ga. Comp. R. & Regs.* r. 272-2-.07 (2004); Indiana, 410 *Ind. Admin.*

Code r. 16-21-1 (1982–2004); Kansas, *Kan. Admin. Regs.* 28-52-2, *Kan. Stat. Ann.* §§ 65-4922–4923 (2003); Kentucky, *Ky. Rev. Stat. Ann.* §§ 216B.155, 216B.165 (2003), Maryland, 10 *Md. Regs. Code.* § 07.01.25 (repealed); Massachusetts, 105 *Code of Mass. Regs.* § 130.331; New Jersey, 8 *N.J. Admin. Code* § 43G-5.6 (2004); New York, *N.Y. Pub. Health Law* § 2805-m (2001); North Carolina, 21 *N.C. Admin. Code* r. 46.1414 (2001); Ohio, *Ohio Admin. Code* §§ 4731-15-02, 4731-15-04 (2003); Pennsylvania, 28 *Pa. Code* § 51.3 (2004) (the provisions of 28 *Pa. Code* § 51.3[f] and [g] [relating to notification] shall be abrogated with respect to a medical facility upon the reporting of a serious event, incident, or infrastructure failure pursuant to § 313; see 40 *P.S.* § 1303.313); Rhode Island, 1956 *R.I. Gen. Laws* § 23-17-40 (2003); South Carolina, 61-16 *S.C. Code of Regs.* § 2-206.2 (these regulations have likely been repealed); South Dakota, *S.D. Codified Laws* § 1-43-19 (1994); Tennessee, *Tenn. Code Ann.* § 63-6-228 (2003); Utah, *Utah Code Ann.* §§ 26-33a-106–107 (2003); Washington, *Wash. Rev. Code* § 70.41.200 (1995) (amended Wash. Legis. Serv., Ch. 145 [SSB 6210], 2004).

8. Alabama and Minnesota.
9. See *Ariz. Admin. Code* R9-20-101.72, R9-20-202; 61-16 *S.C. Code of Regs.* § 2-206.2; *S.D. Codified Laws* § 1-43-19 (1994).
10. See 410 *Ind. Admin. Code* rr. 15-2.2-1, 16.2-3.1-13 (2004).
11. See Ohio Admin. Code § 4731-15-02 (2003).
12. See Ky. Rev. Stat. Ann. §§ 216B.155, 216B.165 (2003).
13. See California Senate Bill (CA SB) 1875 (2000); Conn. Legis. Serv., Public Act 01-145 (SHB 6941) (2001); *Ga. Comp. R. & Regs.* r. 272-2-.07 (2004); 105 *Code of Mass. Regs.* § 130.331; Minnesota Senate File (SF) 560).
14. See *Fla. Admin. Code Ann.*, r. 59a-10.0055 (2004).
15. See 21 *N.C. Admin. Code* r. 46.1414 (2001); 28 *Pa. Code* § 51.3 (2004).
16. See *Colo. Rev. Stat.* § 25-1-124 (2004); *Ohio Admin. Code* § 4731-15-0 (2003).
17. States requiring that the reportable information be forwarded to the state health department or related body include Arkansas, California, Colorado, Indiana, Mississippi, Pennsylvania, Rhode Island, South Carolina, South Dakota, and Utah.
18. States requiring internal institutional reporting include Kansas, Maryland, Minnesota, Ohio, and Washington.

References

American Society for Healthcare Risk Management. [http://www.ashrm.org]. 2004.

Brennan, T. A., and others. "Incidence of Adverse Events and Negligence in Hospitalized Patients: Results from the Harvard Medical Practice Study I." *New England Journal of Medicine*, 1991, *324*, 370–376.

Joint Commission on Accreditation of Healthcare Organizations. "Sentinel Event Policy and Procedures." [http://www.jcaho.org/accredited+organizations/laboratory+services/sentinel+events/index.htm#1]. July 2002.

Kohn, L. T., Corrigan, J. M., and Donaldson, M. S. (eds.). *To Err Is Human: Building a Safer Health System.* Washington, D.C.: National Academies Press, 2000.

Timothy Laubach et al. v. Franklin Square Hospital, 79 Md. App. 203, 556 A.2d 682 (1989), *affm'd.* 318 Md. 615, 569 A.2d 693 (1990).

Livotte v. New York City Health and Hospitals Corporation, West Law 260217 (S.D. N.Y. 1989).

Frank Reyes et al. v. Meadowlands Hospital Medical Center, Superior Court of New Jersey, No. HUD-L-2996-00 (2001).

CHAPTER EIGHT

CLAIMS MANAGEMENT RISKS IN PATIENT SAFETY EVENTS

Pamela L. Popp

The occurrence of a patient safety event, or adverse event, logically will focus the hospital risk manager's attention on the needs of the patient and on the communications to the patient and family about the event and the implications of the plan of care. Unfortunately, this focus can be too narrow, as a multitude of other areas need to be considered in the first few hours after a patient safety event is identified.

The Ripple Effect of a Patient Safety Event: Malpractice, Regulatory Scrutiny, and Potential Fraud and Abuse Litigation

Once the patient's immediate care needs are addressed after an adverse event, the risk manager needs to identify a plan of action to address these other issues:

- Possible malpractice litigation
- State and federal regulatory compliance
- JCAHO compliance
- Billing (potential fraud and abuse implications)
- Staffing
- Information gathering under available privileges (discussed in Chapters Seven and Eleven)

It may be helpful to develop a chart that lays out the time frame for addressing each of these action areas, who needs to be involved, and the privilege that might apply (see the example in Table 8.1).

To illustrate the various factors involved in dealing with claims management risk, this chapter will consider the following basic fact scenario from many angles: a nurse inadvertently administers the wrong drug; the patient goes into cardiac arrest and dies.

Malpractice Litigation Analysis: Is There Liability Exposure?

When contemplating medical malpractice litigation and the organization's liability exposure, the risk manager, along with the defense counsel, needs to fully investigate the cause of the event to determine whether a liability exposure exists for the facility. This is different from the systems focus approach of a root cause analysis. Here there are areas of responsibility that likely will attach to individuals and their actions. The intention here is not to lay blame but instead to determine liability, hold conversations with the involved staff members both as a group (to discuss the process in which the failure occurred, their roles, and the need for communication with counsel) and as individuals (to discuss specific actions that may have led or actually did lead to the event itself). Using a team approach with outside defense counsel guarantees that all conversations and findings are protected by attorney-client privilege.

In our basic scenario the hospital is likely to be exposed to liability simply because the nurse, as a hospital employee, had a duty to the patient to administer the correct medication. She did not do this, and it directly resulted in injury to the patient. Duty, breach of that duty, causation, and injury are needed for a finding of negligence in a courtroom.

State Compliance Analysis: What Needs to Be Reported and When?

The patient's death will trigger several local and state reports, depending on the hospital's location and licensing requirements. At a minimum the hospital should report the event to the medical examiner or coroner (because it involves an unexpected death) and to the state under any applicable state reporting requirements (at the time of this writing, at least twenty four states required event reporting. This could result in an autopsy or other medical examiner (or criminal) investigation. In addition, if licensed individuals are involved, the facility may have an obligation to report the event to the applicable licensing board. This content of this report will be specific to the event and should be handled very carefully by the

TABLE 8.1. MANAGING PATIENT SAFETY EVENT ISSUES: SAMPLE CHART.

Area	Tasks	Privilege	Timeline	Lead Personnel	Identify
Malpractice litigation	Interview staff Copy medical record	Attorney-client	As soon as litigation anticipated	Defense counsel	Liability exposure
State compliance	Prepare notification summary & submit to state	State specific	State specific	Risk manager	Compliance with state notification statutes
JCAHO compliance	Complete root cause analysis process	State specific	45 days	Risk manager or patient safety officer	Compliance with JCAHO standards
Billing	Halt all billings Review bills for appropriate charges Reimburse Medicare or Medicaid if needed	None	Immediate, with refund to federal programs within 45 days	Billing supervisor	Appropriate billings to patient and insurers
Staffing	Talk with staff on behavioral issues Document personnel matters Suspend or terminate staff as needed Arrange staff support if needed	None	Immediate	HR manager	Staff needing support or disciplinary actions

facility reporter. Often, presenting an action plan for the employee's rehabilitation (including training, reassignment, and the like) with the initial reporting will reduce the extent of the state investigation into the individual's acts. If a hearing is needed on the state licensing board report, it is highly recommended that the employee(s) have representation. If the hospital's carrier or self-insurance program allows, it is best if this representation is undertaken by a lawyer who specializes in malpractice defense. This makes it more likely that the information conveyed by the employee in this discoverable setting will be protected and will be consistent with the hospital's malpractice defense strategy should malpractice litigation ensue.

JCAHO Compliance Analysis: What System Failures Contributed to the Event? What Action Plans Will Prevent Reoccurrence?

A root cause analysis of the event should be commenced as soon as possible, with the result completed in forty-five days, because this event qualifies as a *sentinel event* under JCAHO standards, owing to the unexpected death of the patient following the administration of a wrong medication.

Convene the appropriate personnel to complete the root cause analysis, and document the various stages of the analysis. Evaluate systems in this process: How did the medication get to the nurse? Was it entered incorrectly in the ordering process? Was it transcribed incorrectly? Was it a verbal order without reconfirmation? Make an effort to identify the various holes in the process that allowed the event to occur.

Depending on the provisions of the applicable state quality or peer review statutes, specific protections could apply to the results of the root cause analysis and the investigatory process. The risk manager is encouraged to check with defense counsel to identify the appropriate method of protecting these meeting proceedings and findings from subsequent disclosure.

Billing (Potential Fraud and Abuse) Analysis: Are the Charges Appropriate for Quality Care Rendered?

When an adverse event has occurred, facilities accepting federal funding through Medicare or Medicaid should be particularly careful not to bill for certain charges until after a thorough review of all charges has been made, to be sure that only quality care is reflected in those charges. In our scenario, charges for the patient's care up to the time of the incorrect drug administration would be appropriate; but charges for the incorrect medication or for the following code and care would need to be held and not billed to either Medicare or Medicaid. If bills have been sent in error or before the risk manager has time to intercept them, the hospital should arrange for a refund to Medicare or Medicaid as soon as this billing is discovered, advising Medicare or Medicaid that charges were erroneously submitted. In a situation less serious than our scenario, it is often advisable to hold the bill until after disclosure has been made to the patient about the event and its impact on the patient's care. When any adverse occurrence is identified and a decision is being made whether to continue to bill the patient's insurer or the patient, the facility should consider strongly the impact of any collections efforts if the care rendered was unsatisfactory or if patient safety was compromised during the hospitalization.

Having a facility or corporate policy in place allows these billing issues to be discussed and thoroughly researched before a decision is needed following a patient safety event. That policy should include the process for communicating the hold on the bill, the authority levels needed to hold or waive charges, and a procedure for reviewing billing charges in relation to quality requirements.

Staffing Analysis: Were Policies and Procedures Followed Appropriately? Was the Chain of Command Used? Do Any Staff Need Retraining or Counseling?

Often the immediate reaction to a scenario such as the one used here is that the employee who made the error is terminated, without regard to the potential ramifications. If an employee has made a mistake, training should be implemented to prevent its reoccurrence. If a system has failed, the employee needs to be assured that he or she remains valuable to the organization. Often the staff member at the center of the event becomes the most valuable witness for the facility if the matter proceeds to trial in a malpractice case. But if that person is terminated or suspended, he or she often is no longer loyal to the facility or helpful with the defense of the underlying matter. Terminated employees become frustrated witnesses and tend to identify other reasons for the error. Understaffing, budget shortages, management changes, financial restrictions, shortages of supplies, and so on may be identified as not just playing a part in this event but as causal issues and may sound believable to a jury.

Employees should understand that they are important to the facility and that making errors only makes them human. They should be reassured by being informed about any available insurance coverage should the matter proceed into litigation, or legal representation or assistance if the state licensing board investigates their license in response to the matter.

Managing Legal Counsel with Different Needs and Types of Expertise

The management of litigation that employs outside legal counsel is one of the risk manager's more challenging responsibilities. There are times when the risk manager feels solicited, insulted, cajoled, and misunderstood by outside counsel, particularly when the risk manager does not have the benefit of a legal education. Nonetheless it is possible to develop a system to deal with all counsel so one can focus on the essential aspects of the litigation. This is particularly important when the risk manager needs to involve counsel in the early investigation of patient safety issues in order to protect the investigation under the attorney-client privilege.

When undertaking selection of counsel, the risk manager needs to do an internal needs assessment, answering the following questions with information specific to the facility:

- How many defense firms are needed?
- What outcome is desired: trial or settlement?
- Should counsel be aggressive or assertive?
- What relationships already exist at the facility?
- What is (or should be) the settlement reputation of each firm?

Even though the risk manager may feel that he or she knows the answers to most of these questions, it might be best to discuss them in a roundtable session with the leadership of each firm, including the chief executive officer, chief financial officer, and chief medical officer. This will allow the risk manager to gain the perspectives of these persons and also make sure that his or her own expectations and assumptions are in line with those of the administrative personnel.

At the same time as the internal needs assessment is being conducted, the risk manager should develop an outline stating the expectations of the law firms on such issues as billing (amounts and frequency), the involvement of senior lawyers (versus the assignment of inexperienced counsel), the thoroughness and frequency of reporting (monthly or quarterly), and general communication needs (do insurance carriers also need to be in the loop?). Put these expectations into a formal set of counsel guidelines, which will serve as the baseline for the behaviors that the facility expects to receive from its counsel and as a guide for documenting procedural issues (reimbursement for in-house copies, travel costs, overhead, and so forth). These guidelines also may outline resolution procedures, possibly including an arbitration clause, for disputes that may arise during the representation.

The guidelines should address, in clear language, not only the expectations the facility has of counsel but also the responsibilities of internal staff in working with counsel. They also should incorporate the organization's values and mission statement and any policy statements that reflect the organization's perspective on such topics as diversity, religious views, political affiliations, or other qualifying characteristics.

Out of these guidelines also may fall benchmarks by which to evaluate continuing relationships with different law firms. Reserves compared to financial result, the number of days that a file is open, cases sorted by type of occurrence, and average fees—all are possible areas for measurement. In addition the risk manager may desire to do an annual survey of the counsel's "customers" on the services provided by counsel. The survey might collect feedback from the various staff members involved with counsel during the year, with ratings on skill level, preparedness, client knowledge, and law knowledge, among other areas. It is recommended that any feedback be shared with counsel in order to give the firm a chance for improvement or recognition for a job well done.

It also may be possible to establish areas of standardization in defenses, maintaining a database or resource of these areas in order to avoid "reinventing the wheel" for each defense. These defenses might include those involving corporate entities, ownership interests, or specialized areas of practice in the hospital (defenses focused on obstetrics cases, for example). The more standardized information that can be retained in a database for easy reference and provided to defense counsel, the more efficient both counsel and risk manager will be. With our growing technological abilities, it might be possible to scan documents into a database that could then be accessed directly by law firms in response to interrogatory requests or requests for production (this would be particularly important where a corporate entity is involved, because multivenue production requests must have identical responses). Although such a project may seem overwhelming at first, the risk manager should feel comfortable asking his or her primary law firm to start this database, as most firms already use an internal document management system and could input the facility documents easily until a more permanent solution is undertaken. Sample documents to include in such a database might be procedural manuals, JCAHO survey results, administrative or personnel files (of the specific individuals in question), state or federal survey results, inspection records (of the site or issue in question), and anything else that exists in hard copy form and is likely to need to be produced on a regular basis.

Once completed, the guidelines and benchmarks should be shared with counsel candidates so that they have the opportunity to review them, share comments and suggestions, and where necessary, to decline representation. It is imperative that expectations the facility has of outside counsel are clear from the onset of the relationship. Otherwise, it truly will become a risk manager's nightmare trying to control several firms that are not following a standardized plan for communication, billing, or representation. It should be understood that some firms may decline representation because of the direction and strength of management outlined in the guidelines. The risk manager should honor this request and seek other firms if necessary. In some instances, however, concerns can be addressed with revisions to the guidelines as the relationship develops.

Once the internal needs assessment is completed and the risk manager feels confident that he or she understands the type of counsel needed to meet the facility's goals, the risk manager should commence interviews with various firms. For each firm, the risk manager will want to ask

- Who are the proposed team members?
- What coverage or depth of seniority exists at the firm?
- What special skills and education exist?
- How many cases were taken to verdict in the past five years?
- What other accomplishments did the firm members achieve?
- What other entities are represented by this firm?
- Could there be conflicts of representation?
- If there is a conflict, which party will counsel represent?
- Are the firm's internal hierarchical structures equitable?

As an alternative to a panel interview process, a worksheet may be completed for each of the firms, assigning values to the various criteria in order to establish evidence of an objective selection process.

Two to three firms should be selected to handle the various matters likely to come up for the facility, unless the facility exceeds an estimated sixty new legal cases per year. Using several firms allows conflicts to be addressed, joint representations to be handled, and firms to be offered cases that mesh with their areas of specialization. In addition, it encourages a healthy competition between the firms and exposes the risk manager to various personalities, work styles, and viewpoints. This is particularly valuable in complex issues cases, where it may be necessary to retain several of the firms on the same case, for representation of individual providers as well as of the health care facility or corporate structure. When unique representation needs occur (if, for example, unionization at the facility is a factor), it may be necessary to hire specialized firms to handle them rather than relying on general medical malpractice counsel. Some malpractice firms also will have experience in more general practice areas, and will have no problem assisting the facility on these matters; others will be content to stay in the malpractice realm and leave the complex corporate issues to other counsel.

Once the firms are hired, the risk manager is encouraged to set up semiannual meetings with each of the firms. Meeting participants can review all pending matters quickly and make sure that both sides are receiving the information necessary to make strong, joint decisions about the management of the litigation. When setting up each meeting, ask that all counsel who work on the facility matters be present, so that all questions that arise can be addressed immediately.

The key to effective litigation management is staying on top of all pending matters without allowing any one matter to consume all of one's time. To achieve this the risk manager must have confidence in the defense team members and in the process. To build this trust the risk manager may want to communicate extensively with counsel in the initial stages of the relationship. As the relationship grows, more work can be done through informal means, such as electronic communications, support staff communications, and even extension of authority levels (in the form of either taking specific steps in a file or having actual settlement authority). Thus the frequency of meetings with outside counsel will be determined by the number and complexity of the matters assigned to those counsel.

Managing the Needs of Internal Information Users

The increasing focus on data and the increasing use of technology can be an explosive combination when the information being shared is confidential or privileged. It is imperative that the risk manager understands, and at times manages, the flow within the facility of information that contains patient safety event facts.

The first step is to have an established process in the medical records department for the immediate copying, and securing, of the medical record of any patient involved in a significant event. The copy is given to the risk manager so that he or she has a complete picture of the patient's care and treatment. This allows the risk manager to oversee any necessary interventions, such as communicating with the patient or the family or establishing effective communication among the members of the caregiver team to ensure collaboration in the ongoing care.

The medical record of each patient should always be treated with the utmost respect, for it is both a medical chronology and a legal document. If late notations need to be made in any chart, medical record personnel should supervise the entry, to be sure that other portions of the completed chart are not removed or revised. In the instance of a litigated matter, more dramatic measures may need to be undertaken, such as moving the file to a more secure location (without affecting access by any providers rendering care to the patient). As for the archiving of medical records, the risk manager should have good knowledge of any contracting company that has responsibility for copying, transferring to microfiche, or digitizing any medical records. The contract with that company should contain strong indemnification and hold-harmless language that addresses instances in which a medical record is lost, inadvertently released, or miscopied. In addition, the quality of the company's work (and its turnaround time) should be evaluated each year. Feedback from outside counsel and insurance carriers should be solicited to be sure that their needs are being met by the company. This is particularly important when an exclusive contract is involved, which may make decreases in service or quality more likely to occur.

The risk manager also should take an interest in data such as incident reports, sentinel event root cause analyses, claim information, legal files, and loss runs from insurance companies. Although limited privilege may attach to some of these documents (in some jurisdictions, peer review or quality assurance statutes may give protection), these data still should circulate only among those personnel who truly have a need to know them. In most situations, educational efforts, management oversight, and policy compliant reporting all can be done with aggregated information, without the concern of breaching patient confidentiality.

When a significant patient safety event occurs, the risk manager may wish to set up a master file of the pertinent pieces of information and log that information into a database for ease of tracking. This can prevent inadvertent release of patient information and can provide a central location for original documents. For example, the risk manager might obtain the original incident report, root cause analysis, claim letter, and lawsuit documents on an unanticipated patient death and secure them in his or her office until a time when the information can be safely returned to other locations. In some jurisdictions it might be best to locate this repository in defense counsel's offices, where the information can be easily scanned into a database for access by other parties while the originals remain safely secured.

Dealing with Whistle-Blower Situations in Patient Safety Events

When investigating patient safety events, the risk manager should be particularly sensitive to those employees who might feel the need to seek management's immediate attention to an issue or problem rather than waiting for that problem to be addressed through such time-intensive channels as root cause analysis and litigation investigation. Employees need to feel that their concerns are warranted and are understood within the management structure, so that they do not feel the need to take those concerns elsewhere. Open forums for involved personnel, where they are free (without getting into the specifics of a particular event) to brainstorm ideas for improving a process or environment should be encouraged. Facilitators of these conversations should be coached carefully so that they can avoid discussions of event specifics in this nonprivileged setting and instead focus the discussion on quality improvement activities or procedural changes to enhance productivity.

What would motivate a loyal employee to blow the whistle on his or her employer in regard to fraud or other dangerous issues? Employees who feel that their concerns, especially those being taken up through hierarchical channels, are not being addressed sufficiently often will seek outside audiences. These audiences may include the government (for fraud issues), licensure agencies (for clinical issues), and even a plaintiff's attorneys (where the employee feels that caregivers were not honest with a patient or family). Particularly in the case of an unanticipated death or other serious unanticipated outcome, employees may be dealing with their own feelings of helplessness or frustration as well as with the feelings of the patient and family.

It is crucial for the health care organization to put a structure in place that allows employees to express their concerns, anonymously if they wish. This can be an 800 number, a hotline, or a means of contacting ethics personnel trained in obtaining information and investigating without rendering judgment. The facility must provide feedback about these concerns to the employee body in general, indicating that concerns have been heard, identifying changes made in procedures or management in response to concerns, and setting ways for any unresolved issues to be addressed. Frequently, this approach is most successful when the personnel involved are located outside the human resource department, so that employees have less cause to worry that the organization will retaliate against those who raise a concern.

In addition, ensure that after the initial conversations with employees involved in the incident have been held, a support procedure remains in place that allows employees to share additional concerns or suggestions as they work through the event personally and professionally. The risk manager might encourage supervisors and managers to spend more time talking with involved employees or to schedule formal meetings to address outstanding issues. If an employee seems unable or unwilling to share concerns in these settings, he or she should be referred to the facility's employee assistance program, yet another setting in which he or she may convey thoughts and concerns confidentially.

Dealing with Complex Legal Risk Exposure and Coordinated Defense Strategies

It is not unusual for multiple layers of fact finding to occur and for defense theory to develop as information is gathered from surveys, investigations, and possibly malpractice litigation. Often multiple parties are involved in these matters, each working diligently to resolve issues within his or her realm. However, it is imperative that the members of this collective group coordinate their efforts in order to prevent duplication, strive for consistency, and achieve the most efficient and effective outcomes.

Take the example of a medical incident that results in the death of a patient in an emergency room. In a situation where the facility is cited by the state or federal surveying entities for a potential violation of the Emergency Medical Treatment and Labor Act (EMTALA), it is likely that counsel will be hired to work with the facility to reduce exposure and craft new procedures and policies in order to prevent a reoccurrence. In addition, malpractice counsel may be retained to address the discovery commencing in the resulting malpractice case. It also is possible that allegations are being made against the facility as a corporate entity. It then requires corporate counsel representation, in addition to the separate representation for providers named individually (or prevented by conflict from joint representation) in the litigation. Regardless of the identities of the various players, it is imperative that the collective defense group meet at the beginning of the process to outline both individual responsibilities and goals and the overall goals for the group. In this instance the overall goals for the facility will be the reduction (or prevention) of an EMTALA violation and resultant fine. Individual goals for counsel might be the effective defense of their individual defendant while keeping a focus on the development of new procedures and processes to eliminate reoccurrences of the violation.

Once the legal and patient safety issues are resolved, it is a good idea to have counsel jointly hold an educational program for the involved facility staff (likely the emergency room staff in this example) so they can talk with counsel about how the event was handled, what new procedures are in place, and how the situation was (in general terms) resolved. This helps staff achieve closure on the issue and gives them the opportunity to interact with counsel in a positive setting, which may result in increased cooperation in the future if they find themselves working with the same counsel in another litigated matter.

It may be possible for multiple defendants (such as a hospital and a physician and a nurse from that hospital) to be represented by the same outside defense counsel. This can occur only where there is no conflict of interest either in the development of the facts or in the defense theory used for each of the individual care providers. If there is a conflict of any kind, separate counsel should be assigned to each provider (pursuant to the conflict), with the understanding by the various counsel retained that the providers still will undertake a united defense. That simply means that counsel will meet and agree on a few main defense theories to pursue during the litigation, focusing the case on a set of consistent facts, defense theories, and goals. This prevents the various providers from taking positions (most typically in testimony in depositions or during the trial) contrary to the other positions, essentially creating the plaintiff's case instead of staying focused on the defense case. In some venues a united or joint defense agreement, when placed in writing, allows the defendants to share in discovery and strategy without those conversations or interactions being discoverable to the plaintiff attorney. In other venues such conversations would be discoverable and therefore should be conducted only in a protected forum. Outside counsel can advise you about the suitability of specific venues.

Effects of Disclosure on Claims Strategies and Litigation

Disclosure to patients of medical errors and near misses is the most recent imperative given to the health care industry by the Joint Commission on Accreditation of Healthcare Organizations (JCAHO). How disclosure is done, what impact it may have on the culture of the organization and on the patient directly, and how it may affect future malpractice litigation are all areas of concern for the health care provider and facility. Responding to consumer and government pressure (especially the delivery of the first Institute of Medicine report on medical error, *To Err Is Human*, in December 1999), JCAHO added to its survey standards a requirement that each facility have a policy of full disclosure to its patients of *unanticipated outcomes* as well as *near misses*. Although a survey of those policies was anticipated for July 1, 2002, it was delayed in light of the overwhelming response from the health care industry advising that tracking and educating patients on near misses would be almost impossible.

Nonetheless it is now imperative that each health care facility and each physician practice commence the development and implementation of a disclosure policy. The policy should include a *statement of the need and willingness of the patient and physician to have an open and honest relationship, with a constant dialogue between them on the patient's care, treatment, and general health and well-being.* When this philosophy is stated clearly in the policy, it becomes the guiding principle for the conversations that follow. The complete policy should be conveyed through in-service programs to all applicable staff, so that these communication needs can be recognized when a patient directs questions or concerns to personnel other than his or her treating physician. The policy should also state *who is responsible for primary communication to the patient when an unanticipated outcome, treatment plan change, or other important information must be communicated.* In most instances the responsible person should be the primary treating physician, because patients want to hear from their physician when it comes to important information (including negative information) about their health and treatment plans. This holds true even in an emergency or surgical situation, where the patient may not have a true relationship with the involved physician but still will want to have him or her as the primary source of treatment information. Because it is the physician's clinical judgment that sets the plan of treatment for the patient, the physician is seen as the most credible of the care-givers when patients are looking for information. In addition the policy should outline *who is responsible for documentation in the patient's record and what should be docu-mented when a disclosure conversation takes place with a patient or family member.* The doc-umentation, like all medical record documentation, should be objective, complete, and accurate. For disclosure conversations, it should state who was present for the conversation, what information was conveyed, what questions were asked by the patient (and what answers were given by the physician), and the agreed-upon next steps in the patient's plan of treatment.

Patient Communication

The issue of who is responsible for patient communication has always been an area of dispute in the hospital environment, often with significant turf battles taking place between nurses and physicians. Where the nurses may feel obligated to over-communicate with the patient, often the physicians are found to undercommuni-cate. The nurses' perspective may be more advocative, social, and interactive, the physicians' more science-based and impersonal. Often this does not cause a problem in the patient's care or treatment. However, when an error or medical misadventure occurs, this communication imbalance can be one of the deciding factors when a patient or family pursues litigation against the providers and entity.

Done correctly, negative disclosure to the patient should be open, honest, and limited to the information truly known. Often the patient's condition will be known before the cause or event sequence is identified, and therefore the communica-tions to the patient should be limited to this information. Speculation, on the cause, fault, or even outcome, is never beneficial. Instead the health care provider should give the patient *the information he or she needs to understand what is happening in the treat-ment plan, why any changes have taken place in that plan, and what to be aware of in the form of reactions or consequences.* This way patients have enough information to ap-preciate how the situation affects them but do not have enough information to shift their focus to external forces or blame. This allows patients to make informed decisions on treatment plan changes and to take appropriate levels of responsi-bility for communicating any changes in their condition to the providers.

The disclosure conversation should take place in the patient's room, with the attending physician leading the conversation, if possible. If this is not possible, then a provider with whom the patient has developed a relationship should begin the conversation, explaining to the patient that something unexpected has occurred, that the outcome will be controlled as best as possible, and that the patient's treatment and care are of the utmost concern. Only when the patient's immediate concerns about care and treatment are resolved should the caregiver proceed to answer any questions about the process or system that allowed the error. Oftentimes it is sufficient to simply explain to the patient that the matter (the cause or system failure) will be investigated and appropriate changes made but that the immediate concern is the *patient's* safety and well-being.

Done incorrectly, disclosure becomes simply an admission of liability and immediately places the situation in a litigious posture. It shifts the focus from the patient's condition, treatment plan, or concerns to the blame of an individual or process. This is of benefit to no one and may even cause subtle reactions or changes in the patient's care to be missed due to distraction on the part of the providers and the patient.

Litigation from Disclosure

It is unrealistic to think that every disclosure conversation will go as well as planned, and that malpractice litigation will never result from properly disclosed errors or occurrences. Nonetheless, without the disclosure conversation, litigation would seem to be more likely, because oftentimes the primary factor in a patient's decision to pursue a malpractice case is lack of communication from the provider on an unexpected outcome or undesirable result. Knowing this, one could speculate that having *any* conversation with the patient might decrease the chance of litigation and alleviate concerns (emotional, psychological, or financial) and thus potentially *prevent* litigation.

In situations where litigation still does occur, the disclosure conversation will be crucial to the trial strategy formation. What was said, how it was documented, and who was present will all be key facts to consider and analyze once litigation is filed. It should not be assumed that a jury will perceive a disclosure conversation immediately as being an admission. Instead, the defense should use the conversation, the providers' concern, and the information shared as a key advantage. Why may the fact that a disclosure occurred work on behalf of the defense in court? Because it meets the *expectations* of the jurors. Jurors feel that there should be an admission when there is a medical error or mistake, whether or not the error or mistake resulted in any harm to the patient. The disclosing provider has immediate credibility before the jury and indeed may become a key witness at trial for the defense.

Conclusion

Organizations that have practiced open disclosure approaches with their patients have found that it actually decreases their litigation. Often the conversation with the patient results in a small bill waiver or facilitation of another medical resource (a continued stay, social services, or discharge planning, for example) to resolve the patient's resulting medical condition. Once these concerns are resolved, the patient no longer has the incentive to pursue litigation against the providers or facility. In fact, over the years, children's hospitals have found this to be the case across the country, simply because children's hospital providers often spend much more time communicating with concerned parents over their child's condition than a physician in an acute setting may spend discussing a care or treatment plan with an adult patient.

A culture of disclosure does not need to be seen as a new fad or requirement. Instead it can be viewed as confirmation of an already existing culture of patient autonomy, honesty, and informed consent. Presenting the disclosure policy as something new can raise staff and provider suspicions that the motivation for the facility is solely litigation prevention or mitigation. Instead, providers need to be reassured that the facility has always encouraged free patient communication and that stating this view in a formal policy at this time is to demonstrate its existence to JCAHO and to provide an outline for its consistent application.

CHAPTER NINE

FULL DISCLOSURE

James R. Woods Jr.

The heart of medical care is communication. Unlike the mathematical field of engineering, medicine always has been more an art than a science. Despite the advances in technology that threaten to intervene between care provider and patient, the essence of medical care remains two parties, the patient and the care provider, working together to resolve a medical challenge. Essential to that working relationship is effective communication. But how does a care provider convey risk in the course of informed consent? How does communication reinforce patient safety and quality care? What does a patient hear? How does he or she factor these risks into a decision for treatment? And what does the care provider say when an unanticipated event occurs?

Historically, the need for honest, forthright communication was driven more by the personalities of the care provider and the patient than by outside forces demanding that effective communication be maintained between these two parties. For the generation of patients now over sixty-five years old, it was atypical to challenge the physician. To this day, many of that generation find it uncomfortable to bother the physician on a weekend or at night. That cannot be said of the younger generation of patients who are comfortable with questioning medical care and challenging decisions that have been made.

Where Does the Education Begin?

Today's medical schools are recognizing the importance of teaching the art form of communication formally. Classes in many medical schools are constructed to introduce communication skills. Standard patient volunteers are employed as surrogate patients so that medical students can try out these skills. Young care providers, however, seldom have experienced traumatic events in their lives, and the ability of the young care provider to understand what it is like to be on the other side of the conversation is weakened by this lack of life experience. Of course in time the young care provider will age and undoubtedly will experience some of life's crises. A spouse may die of breast cancer, a child may develop a life-threatening infection, or the physician may be sued and thus fear professional licensure actions or the loss of his or her economic stability.

Another reason why communication is such a difficult task for young care providers is their fear about what to say and how the patient will respond. Upon receiving adverse information will the patient become silent or suddenly scream out and verbally or even physically attack the care provider? This angst is present even when the care provider feels that he or she has not done anything improper. It becomes more intense when the medical issues fall in gray areas. Whether to order a test is often determined not by biology but by the attitude held by the care provider at that moment. Tests that are indicated for obvious reasons offer no dilemma. It is that test that might have been ordered but was deferred that haunts the care provider if in fact a bad outcome occurs that was predictable with that test. If risks associated with their care were explained to patients as part of informed consent, patients' need for explanations of unanticipated outcomes would diminished markedly. This point has been reiterated in the literature on the subject of consent to treatment (Rozovsky, 2003) and unanticipated disclosure (Woods and Rozovsky, 2003).

The Art of Describing Risk

The language we use to educate our patients before a surgical or medical procedure is subject to the challenges of obtaining informed consent. Examples of expressions heard frequently in medical offices or on hospital wards are

"It's very unlikely to happen."

"I've never personally seen it."

"If it happened, it would be a case report."

"We're going to do everything we can to avoid it."

"Don't worry."

Influential in this process of communicating risk is the attitude and experience of the presenter (care provider) and the educational level and expectations of the receiver (patient) of this information.

How Do Patients Perceive Risk?

A number of factors influence the way in which risk is perceived (Laudan, 1994; Adams and Smith, 2001; Lloyd, 2001; Lloyd, Hayes, Bell, and Naylor, 2001; Woods, 2004). These factors are better understood when risk is related to societal events than when it is linked to medical treatments or procedures.

Risks appear greater when they are inconceivable and less when they seem commonplace. In December 2003 and January 2004, U.S. newspapers headlines addressed the risk of mad cow disease (bovine spongiform encephalopathy) following the death in Washington state of a cow that presumably originated from a Canadian herd. The risk that an individual in the United States would contract this disease is negligible, especially with the meat-processing laws now in effect. Yet the headlines, not weighing the single cow against the number of people in the United States who eat meat, would lead one to fear that the risk was significant. For another example, recall the headlines focused on terrorism that were on front pages of newspapers throughout the United States as New Year's Eve 2003 approached and the terrorist action warnings rose from yellow to orange. The world was focused on the possibilities of a repeat of the September 11, 2001, attack. Yet for any one individual in the United States, the risk of dying from a terrorist attack was extremely small—especially when contrasted to the risks being taken by the hundreds of thousands of people who were driving to New York City to celebrate New Year's Eve, many of them smoking or drinking alcohol.

Risks that others might incur are interpreted as greater than the risks that might affect the individual. If asked about the chance of being diagnosed with cancer in the next ten years, we likely would estimate it as higher for others, lower for ourselves. This may reflect our optimism or our opinion (correct or incorrect) that we can control our own destiny and environment (through diet or exercise) better than can anyone else. Or we may use denial as a defense that allows us to continue to engage in risk activities that we associate with adverse outcomes, believing that others engaging in the same behaviors are more likely than we are to incur a bad outcome.

What Constitutes Significant Risk and How Should It Be Described?

Risk is a probability. It is calculated as follows:

$$\text{Risk} = \frac{\text{People experiencing an adverse outcome from the activity}}{\text{People engaged in the activity}}$$

To demonstrate this calculation in its simplest form, each of us has a 100 percent risk of dying in our lifetime:

$$\frac{\text{People who are born}}{\text{People who die}} = 100\%$$

We also should distinguish *absolute risk* from *relative risk*. The newspapers, by using absolute risk to describe only part of the story, daily provide examples of how reporting can be biased. A quality assurance report that states, "Thirteen medication errors were detected over a one-month period in Pharmacy X," provides only absolute risk. To be more meaningful, the risk should be expressed as a relative risk: that is, it should be calculated in relation to the total number of medications filled during that same time period. The report has more meaning when it states, "Thirteen medication errors were detected in Pharmacy X in one month in which 4,850 medication transactions occurred."

The significance of risk numbers differs with the individual, the event, and the consequence. In general, any risk judged to be less than 1:1,000,000 is considered insignificant. Here, risk numbers have a way of depersonalizing the impact. If the risk is remote but catastrophic, it might still be very significant. For example, if the risk of death from a general anesthetic is 1 in 100,000, it might seem insignificant until one factors in the type of risk: death. In general, what constitutes a significant risk is a personal decision, and patients do personalize risk. For them, a risk is either 100 percent or 0 percent. The magnitude of risk may be made more understandable if it is quantified in relation to an individual living in a community (Table 9.1) (Calman and Royston, 1997).

Risk may be presented as a percentage: for example, "Two percent of deliveries may end in shoulder dystocia" (Gherman, 2002), Unfortunately, patients tend to comprehend interpretation of percentage of risk poorly. In one study (Beyth-Marom, 1982), a number of individuals were asked to estimate the percentages implied by qualitative terms. They said that

"Certain" meant 98 to 100 percent.

"Can't rule out" meant 24 to 49 percent.

"There is a chance" meant 37 to 60 percent.

TABLE 9.1. RISK QUANTIFIED IN RELATION TO AN INDIVIDUAL LIVING IN A COMMUNITY.

Community	Number	Suggested Qualitative Term
Individual	1	High
Family	10	High
Street	100	Moderate
Village	1,000	Low
Small town	10,000	Very low
Large town	100,000	Minimal
City	1,000,000	Negligible
Country	10,000,000	Negligible

Risk appears greater when described in terms of negative outcomes than when described in terms of positive outcomes. A "70 percent survival" rate is viewed more favorably than a "30 percent mortality" rate, even though their numerical values are the same (Lloyd, 2001). However, a positive correlation exists between degrees of risk and benefit to one's health (Lloyd, Hayes, Bell, and Naylor, 2001).

Rate of risk may be understood by some more clearly than proportions. In one obstetrical study, patients were asked about their understanding of risk for fetal genetic conditions. The data were given either as rates (2.6:1,000 versus 8.9:1,000 women) or proportions (1 in 384 versus 1 in 112 women) (Grimes and Snively, 1999). Rates were better understood (73 percent of participants recognized the differences) than proportions (only 56 percent recognized the differences). Moreover, those better educated scored higher than those with less formal education. In either set of data only 80 percent were able to discriminate which relationship was greater than the other.

Other Precautions in Relaying Risk Information

Risk profiles should take into consideration the individual's behavior, lifestyle, family history, and risk-seeking activities. In most cases, risk profiling should describe baseline risk and then adjust that risk based on the characteristics of the patient himself or herself. In a review of risk for retained instruments or sponges at Brigham and Women's Hospital from 1985 to 2001, higher risks were linked to greater body mass index, emergency rather than elective surgery, and unexpected changes in the type of surgery during the case (Gawande and others, 2003). Yet seldom do surgeons address the possibility of a retained instrument or sponge when they counsel obese patients about the risks of a surgical procedure.

Patients have difficulty recalling exact information given verbally. Thus risks should be given to the patient in writing. In one study, when asked after a counseling session to recall their diagnosis, only 31 percent of individuals could do so accurately (Ellis, Hopkin, Leitch, and Crofton, 1979). Yet 70 percent could do so when the diagnosis was given to them in a written form.

The inability of individuals to recall medical treatments or procedures is reinforced by study results for obstetric patients. Olson and others (1997) cite the results of telephone interviews obtained up to eight years after delivery with 302 patients and 558 matched controls. The interview results were compared with data from the actual medical records. Birth weight and gestational age at delivery were recalled accurately, reproductive medical procedures (amniocenteses and ultrasounds) were moderately recalled, and pregnancy and postpartum complications were poorly recalled. Of note, time from delivery to telephone interview did not affect reliability of recall. More recently, a survey questionnaire of 277 postpartum women administered within months of delivery again documented patients' difficulty recalling medical events. Overall, 60 percent had imperfect recall of events. In this study cohort of 42 percent white, 40 percent black, and 16 percent Hispanic patients, blacks had greater than two times odds of incorrectly recalling one or more events (Elkadry and others, 2003). Had these individuals been given a written report of their care, their recall most likely would have been improved.

Risks should not be personalized by the care provider. When a known risk has not happened to us or to those colleagues we work with, then we tend to deemphasize the risk. It is the old "I've personally never seen it." As a corollary, when we have encountered such an event, irrespective of its rarity, we tend to include it in our counseling about risk outcomes.

Applying These Lessons About Risk to Obtaining Informed Consent

In 1997, Singh and Paling published a tool called the Paling Perspective Scale for Describing Risk. In their easily understood diagram, they described risk prevalence in a logarithmic graph with a range of 10^0 (risk of 1 in 1) to 10^{-12} (risk of 1 in 1 trillion). They then reduced this risk to a simple linear scale of $+6$ to -6. In this graph, 1 in 1 million (noted as zero) was the middle of the scale and risk up to 1 in 10,000 ($+2$) included such events as drowning this year, being killed in an airplane, and dying of cancer from having one light beer per day for one year, but also the risk for women of dying from the birth of a single child. More recently, Stallings and Paling modified their general risk profile to cover only obstetrical

TABLE 9.2. OBSTETRIC AND GYNECOLOGIC RISKS COMPARED WITH GENERAL LIFE RISKS.

Occurrence	Estimate
Drowning in tub this year	1:600,000
Being killed in an airplane crash	1:250,000
Dying from female sterilization	**1:70,000**
Dying of cancer from one light beer/day for one year	1:50,000
Dying from birth of a single child	**1:15,000**
Dying from a cesarean section	**1:11,000**
Trisomy 13	1:11,000
Turner's syndrome	1:10,000
Dying from a lightning strike	1:9,000
Trisomy 18	1:8,000
Dying from vaginal hysterectomy	**1:3,500**
Dying from an ectopic pregnancy	**1:2,500**
Dying from abdominal hysterectomy	**1:1,400**
Ureter injury from vaginal hysterectomy	**1:1,000**
Loss of fetus from amniocentesis	**1:200**
Ureter injury from abdominal hysterectomy	**1:100 to 1:50**
Operative site infection	**1:15**

Source: Adapted from Stallings and Paling, 2001.

and gynecological procedures (Stallings and Paling, 2001). They grouped between 1 in 10,000 and 1 in 10 the risk of events such as mortality from vaginal or abdominal hysterectomy, ureter injuries during a vaginal or abdominal hysterectomy, and operative site infections. Similar charts described the risks of genetic disorders (trisomy 13, 18, Turner's syndrome, and others) and obstetrical mortality (from pregnancy, cesarean section, female sterilization, and so forth). When these obstetrical and gynecological events are compared with general life risks, they provide an overview of risk in medicine (Table 9.2). Time will tell whether patients benefit from this type of approach.

An example that brings out all the dilemma in patients' decision making quite simply may be that of a woman I'll call BJ:

BJ is told that her genetic screening test places her at a 1:200 risk of having a baby with Down's syndrome. However, the means of determining that issue, an amniocentesis for karyotype determination, carries a 1:200 risk of a miscarriage. How does BJ respond to these low risk numbers, and can she place them in the context of her personal life, which is influenced by religious, ethical, moral, and practical factors? As is common in medicine, the description of risk may be the easiest of the issues here. She might be informed that the 1:200 risk attaching to the existence of the genetic condition and to the loss of the pregnancy from amniocentesis is "very small." She might find that risk more understandable if it is described as one individual out of all those living on a street, as compared with one individual out of a family or one out of a medium-sized village. It would not be appropriate to describe either risk in terms of "I have not seen this in my practice." It would be appropriate to acknowledge to BJ that these risks are given as relative numbers based on all amniocenteses and all gathered data about genetic conditions. Both are generic risk figures and may not apply to her specifically. Moreover, either the loss from an amniocentesis or the presence of a genetic condition is all or none when it applies to BJ herself as opposed to the general population. Providing the information as a percentage (0.5 percent) probably offers no advantage over semiquantitative descriptors, but informing her that either 199 out of 200 pregnancies or amniocenteses end in good results may provide reassurance, as compared with informing her that 1 in 200 or 0.5 percent end in an adverse event.

Notwithstanding the importance of providing a clear description of risks, the care provider must be aware that these risks then must be factored into BJ's personal life. In this case the amniocentesis would be judged an elective choice on BJ's part, whereas the outcome of the pregnancy in terms of the risk of a genetic condition in the fetus is not hers to decide. Thinking in these terms, BJ may choose not to take an active role in the decision making but to let events unfold naturally, or she may be one who feels life is a series of choices and may make her choice based on that philosophy. BJ may also view the risk of loss from an amniocentesis as existing at one end of a continuum and the risk of a genetic condition for her fetus as existing at the other end. She then may overlay her personal beliefs onto that continuum. For example, she may know a family who has raised a genetically exceptional child with love and great satisfaction. Or she may know of a family who attempted to raise a genetically exceptional child only to find that the stress led to divorce and disruption of the family unit. Finally, the issues that lead her to make a decision may not be clear to the care provider who tells her the data. She may fear needles and reject an amniocentesis because of the pain she perceives she would experience. She may be under pressure by her partner to end the pregnancy because of his fear of raising a genetically exceptional child.

This example highlights the complexities of presenting seemingly straightforward decision choices based on risks—that is, the risk of pregnancy loss from an amniocentesis versus the risk of a genetically exceptional fetus—and it alerts the care provider to be cognizant of the complexities of such a conversation.

How Do Patients Manage the Risks in Their Decision Making?

Despite a growing body of literature on care providers' communication and patients' perceptions of risk, few studies have addressed what patients do with medical information. One would hope that a patient would consider each component of care, measure risk versus benefit, examine the alternatives for care (and their risks), and then choose a course of management. This seldom happens. Yet patients need help to do just this. Witness the efforts to assist patients to participate in their treatment choices (Whelan and others, 1999, 2003; O'Connor and others, 1999). When they completed a decision tree, patients were more informed, felt less in conflict in their decisions, and were more involved in the final plans than were controls (O'Connor and others, 1999). Use of a decision board among breast cancer patients resulted in improved understanding by the patients and clearer communication by care providers (Whelan and others, 1999, 2003).

Without such aids, patients must still make choices in consenting to treatment, but their method of choosing becomes more vague. The choices they make in this area of vague information can have a negative impact on patient safety. As Lloyd (2001) and Lloyd, Hayes, Bell, and Naylor (2001) have indicated, patients may resort to "short cuts" in order to simplify the process. Thus a lengthy conversation with the care provider is reduced by the patient to only a few items as he or she struggles to make sense of the options. Others resort to a dependency role, as expressed by questions such as, "Doctor, if it were your family member, what would you do?" In the future, students of informed consent must continue to search for tools that enable the patient to sort through options of care, recognize the risks and benefits of each, and choose wisely the path best suited for that individual and his or her family.

How Should We Counsel Patients About Risk?

Even as care providers search for ways to incorporate risk counseling into their approach to informed consent, there appear to be several concepts that we can use immediately in offering risk counseling to patients.

Keep it simple. Patients have a difficult time repeating what they have heard. Write down the important facts and give them to the patient.

Remember that individuals differ in how they understand risk. Use proportions, percentages, rates, and qualitative words (*low, high, likely, certain, cannot be sure*) so the patient does not need to take semiquantifiable or even qualitative words and correlate them accurately with true risk. If possible, state the risk in terms the patient can understand: for example, "This is the equivalent of one person experiencing this risk out of a village of people."

Consider the patient's education. All patients deserve explanations of the risks that are consistent with their understanding. In one study of 681 informed consent forms, computer assessment placed the education required to understand them at the 12.6 grade level. Of 616 surgical consent forms, only 29 could be understood by an individual reading at less than the eighth-grade level. The researchers concluded that most consent forms are too complex to be understood easily by typical patients (Hopper, Tenhave, Tully, and Hall, 1998). Never assume, however, that an individual with higher education will always understand complicated medical descriptions of procedures or treatments.

Do not offer anecdotal risk descriptions. The fact that a care provider encountered an adverse outcome somewhere in his or her training does not change the known risk probability. Nonetheless, risk counseling for invasive procedures must also take into consideration the skills of the operator and the anticipated operating time. Perhaps the most important question is this: Is the risk for this patient greater than that quoted for anyone undergoing this procedure? Answers to that question take into account the skills of the operator, the nature of the operation, and the characteristics of the patient to be operated on.

Understand that the care provider and the patient may see risk differently. For example, the patient who is obese and has Type 1 diabetes, who wants a vaginal delivery, and whose baby is judged to weigh 4,050 grams has a different risk profile for a successful vaginal delivery than does a patient who is slim and does not have diabetes and whose baby is also judged to weigh 4,050 grams. From the patient's standpoint, her risks that result from being obese, a smoker, driving to the hospital, and desiring a vaginal birth (all seemingly low risks in her opinion) may in her mind pale in comparison to her concerns about the duration of labor, risks from an epidural anesthetic, her lack of control during labor, her wish to choose her treatment, and her unspoken fears that her baby may have been affected by her smoking. Because her understanding of how a vaginal delivery for a large baby is carried out is vague, the medical issues in that process may well be low on her list of concerns.

Ask the patient to repeat back the risk information you have given. If the information has been presented clearly, the patient should be able to repeat the risks back to the care provider, in her own terms.

Document the discussion in the medical record. Record the type of data provided to the patient as part of the informed consent process, using the same wording (percentages, proportions, qualitative terms) that was given to the patient.

Are Care Providers Their Own Worst Enemies?

The communication strategies used by care providers with patients can consciously or unconsciously restrict the exchange of ideas. At other times those strategies can become a shield, protecting the care provider from the emotional overtones of the conversation. In a 1984 audiotape study of seventy-four patients seen in a primary care internal medicine practice, after patients were asked what problem brought them to see a doctor, only 23 percent were able to complete their opening statements of concern before being interrupted. The mean duration before the patient was interrupted was eighteen seconds (Beckman and Frankel, 1984). That study was small and focused on a university practice, so a second, larger study was conducted in 1999 (Marvel, Epstein, Flowers, and Beckman, 1999). Two hundred and sixty-four patient-physician interviews, involving twenty-nine board-certified family physicians, were taped at several practice sites in the United State and Canada. In this study, 28 percent of patients completed their initial statements of concern. Those who did not were interrupted at a mean duration of twenty-three seconds. Braddock and others (1999) studied and audiotaped patient encounters with general internists, family practice physicians, and general and orthopedic surgeons. Of 3,552 discussions that led to clear decisions, only 9 percent met all the criteria for complete decision making. Although 71 percent of the proposed interventions were discussed, only 1.5 percent of these discussions included any effort to assess the patient's understanding. What better evidence of the failure of care providers to involve patients in decision making? Failure to involve patients also may be reflected in a care provider's inability to seek out (or lack of interest in seeking out) direct or indirect comments (*clues*) about personal aspects of the patient's life or evolution. In a study of 116 randomly selected office visits to primary care physicians and surgeons, Levinson, Gorawara-Bhat, and Lamb (2000) found that 70 percent of these personal clues were initiated by the patient and only 30 percent by the physician asking a question. Yet the researchers judged the clues to be a "cry for help."

In a study of the use of slang in medicine (Coombs, Chopra, Schenk, and Yutan, 1993), an extensive review of journals, interviews, and other forms of information was carried out to determine whether in fact the use of medical slang was influenced by the stage of one's medical career. Understandably, premed students and medical students in their first and second years seldom used medical slang. Medical students in years three and four, however, began using medical slang to an increased degree, similar to the usage of residents and faculty in the early stages of their careers. Only as the age of the faculty increased did the need to use slang in communications decrease. When one considers the significance of these findings, it appears that medical slang is used early in one's medical career mostly as a defense, shielding the individual from the seriousness with which he or she now must take the medical profession. With age and personal experience of loss, a care provider's need for and therefore use of slang decreased.

Picture this scenario:

Two residents rotating through the neonatal intensive care nursery are attending a baby severely asphyxic at birth who was delivered the night before. As they take the elevator to the cafeteria for a cup of coffee, they fail to recognize members of the extended family of the newborn who are also in the elevator. One resident says to the other, "You know, that baby delivered last night is CTD." The other resident turns and asks what CTD means. The first resident, in a jocular manner, says, "it means circling the drain." The family members, outraged by this show of insensitivity, immediately call the medical director of that hospital to demand an apology and to indicate the family's utter disgust with the health care system and the level of care provided at that hospital. Despite what may be the highest level of health care provided that newborn and despite the possibility that the condition of that newborn is not a result of human error, this family is now poised to lay a label of malpractice on any small departure from recovery that the newborn may show, even though the residents in the elevator may play no active role in the care provided this newborn. Slang has created a hostile and explosive situation due to the anger and disgust with the health system that the extended family now feels. This situation was unnecessary and possibly detrimental to the support the extended family now can provide to the mother and father of the newborn.

The concept of communicating openly with patients means different things to different care providers. When medical students graduate from medical school they take the Hippocratic oath. Although untold versions of this oath have been written (and most medical schools have modernized the oath for their students), none contains a clear statement regarding fully disclosing information about an unanticipated adverse outcome.

Once a physician has graduated, it is understandable that disclosure should be synonymous with telling the truth. But what does telling the truth in medicine mean? Picture this scenario:

A physician is carrying out a routine cesarean section on a young patient and encounters excessive bleeding. Because her hospital lacks the technology for interventional radiology and embolization, she is forced to do a hysterectomy. After the surgery she addresses the family and explains the events and the reasons for the hysterectomy. Here, disclosure simply means detailing the events while using terms the family can understand.

But if the outcome is adverse, does disclosure mean that the care provider must confess all of his or her thoughts about management steps that in fact were not chosen? Imagine the following:

Your twenty-five-year-old patient, pregnant for her first time, presents to your office at thirty-five weeks' gestation complaining of decreased fetal movement. Your first impulse is to obtain a test to evaluate the status of the fetus. As she sits in your office, however, she acknowledges that her fetus is beginning to kick a little bit, and she seems somewhat reassured. Because you are behind in seeing patients, you choose not to order that test. Unfortunately, she comes into the triage area the next weekend with an intrauterine fetal death. Following delivery, an autopsy is carried out but reveals no cause for the death. In the back of your mind, you wonder whether it would have made a difference if you had ordered that test. Are you obliged to tell the patient that you thought about testing but chose not to do it based on what she said, thereby transferring the responsibility from you to the patient?

What Do Patients Want from Their Care Providers?

A number of studies have been conducted to expose elements of health care that lead to medical malpractice suits. Failure to communicate positions itself at the top of most lists. Hickson, Clayton, Githens, and Sloan (1992) assessed reasons for filing malpractice suits given by 127 families following an adverse perinatal event. Not surprisingly, 43 percent sued because of their feelings that there had been a cover-up or that they should seek revenge. This supports Witman, Park, and Hardin's findings (1996), in a survey of patients seeing an internist, that patients would sue if they discovered unreported moderate to severe mistakes in care. Gallagher and others (2003) studied attitudes of six focus groups of adult patients who encountered medical errors. Disclosure of all harmful errors, the reasons for them, and future preventive steps and receipt of an apology characterized their unmet needs.

Rules About Disclosure

Rules and standards for disclosure are beginning to be addressed in some professional standards, state laws, and policies of individual hospitals.

Professional Standards

National societies have established their own rules for disclosure. On the one hand the American Medical Association's *Code of Medical Ethics* acknowledges that a physician is ethically required to tell the patient if medical care or judgment resulted in a medical complication (AMA, 1997, § 8.12:125; Rosner and others, 2000). Likewise the American College of Physicians' *Ethics Manual* (1998) requires that all information regarding care or intended procedures should be disclosed if that information compromises the patient's well-being.

On the other hand the specialty societies have been reluctant to declare full and open disclosure as a basic principle of care when adverse events occur. The American College of Obstetricians and Gynecologists' *Code of Professional Ethics* (2001) advocates that care providers "deal honestly with patients" but takes no position on disclosing medical practices leading to adverse outcomes. The American Academy of Pediatrics (1996), in a policy statement titled "Ethics and the Care of Critically Ill Infants and Children," addresses the importance of engaging the parents when life-sustaining medical technology is used but takes no position on open disclosure of adverse events.

The Joint Commission on Accreditation of Healthcare Organizations (JCAHO, 2001) has addressed disclosure. Its standard is that "patients and, when appropriate, their families are informed about the outcomes of care, including unanticipated outcomes." Disclosure also has been cited by the American Society for Healthcare Risk Management (ASHRM). In its *Code of Professional Ethics and Conduct*, ASHRM states that one specific obligation care providers must meet is to "communicate and disclose information to patients and, when appropriate, others honestly and factually" (ASHRM, 2001). ASHRM also has published four white papers that amplify the ethical obligation to disclose information to patients regarding adverse and unanticipated outcomes of care (ASHRM, June 2001, 2002, 2003, 2004).

State Laws Protecting Disclosure

State laws now offer some protection to care providers who fully disclose information to the patient when an adverse event occurs. In Colorado, for example, any information that is related to a bad outcome and that conveys sympathy is judged inadmissible as evidence of liability in a civil suit (13 *Colo. Rev. Stat.* 25, 2003). Similar statutes now exist in Texas, California, Florida, and Massachusetts (ASHRM, 2004).

Individual Hospitals' Responsibilities

Individual hospitals now are taking the lead in establishing policies for disclosure. At the University of Rochester Strong Memorial Hospital, the policy (University of Rochester, 2001) reads: "It is the policy to encourage open, ongoing communication with patients about all aspects of their health care and the results of such care. . . . This includes the right to be informed of unanticipated or negative outcomes. . . . The fact that an outcome is unexpected or negative should not cause delay in the patient being advised of the outcome." This policy is, however, balanced by this statement: "It is not appropriate or necessary to admit fault or criticize others when advising the patient of a negative or unanticipated outcome. . . . The focus should be directed toward future management."

Does Full Disclosure Work?

A menu for managing full disclosure following an adverse outcome offers four principles (Kraman and Hamm, 1999). Early injury review should be followed by significant efforts to maintain the patient-institution (hospital) relationship. The outcome then should be disclosed. This should be followed by fair compensation to the family for the injury. Finally, programmatic—or systems—issues require an analysis of events and participants.

To date the body of data demonstrating the effectiveness and cost containment of this level of disclosure is limited. A frequently cited study from a tertiary Veterans Administration system serving 18,000 patients in Lexington, Kentucky, offers some insight (Kraman and Hamm, 1999). From 1990 to 1996, following two substantial malpractice judgments against the system in 1987, a program of full disclosure was instituted, even if the next of kin was unaware that an error had occurred. During that period eighty-eight malpractice claims were made. The results of these claims were then compared with claim expenses for thirty-five similar tertiary veterans medical centers east of the Mississippi. Only five centers had higher claim numbers than the Kentucky facility; yet twenty-eight centers had higher claim settlements.

As noted by Wu (1999), the value of these data outside the VA system remains to be determined. In the private sector average claim settlements are double those in the VA system. Furthermore, the Veterans Administration offers universal free coverage and can offer remedial treatment and eventually disability payments. Moreover, the care providers, as government workers, are protected from personal liability.

Disclosure Strategies

There are basic principles that should always be adhered to when the care provider must disclose elements of the care associated with an adverse outcome. Following these principles enhances patient safety by fostering a framework of open, forthright discussion.

- *Allow adequate time for the conversation.* Disclosing adverse results or explaining an adverse outcome should never be done in a hurry. Although it is unrealistic to leave an indeterminate amount of time for such a conversation, the care provider must recognize the possibility that a conversation may last longer than expected and be prepared to cancel either patient appointments or other activities if the time required to complete the conversation satisfactorily so demands.
- *Identify an appropriate, safe place for the conversation.* At times it may be necessary to have a conversation in the physician's office. That may be comfortable for the patient also. But if returning to the hospital and having the discussion in the doctor's office generates additional irate feelings in the patient, the care provider may choose a location for the conversation that is more neutral and less likely to antagonize the patient.

- *Plan the conversation in advance.* Although the care provider will not have a script during the conversation, it is important that he or she have an idea of the issues that will be raised and an approach for each of those issues. It may be necessary for young care providers to sit with a more seasoned colleague and role-play a conversation before the actual conversation occurs. Alternatively, the care provider may jot down a few phrases that can be used in the conversation.
- *Consider the arrangement of the room in which the conversation will be held.* Some physicians and patients choose a room arrangement with a big desk that separates care provider from care receiver, diplomas on the wall, and bookshelves lined with medical texts. Others prefer that the physician and patient be seated in a simpler room arrangement, perhaps around a small round table, absent the diplomas and books. A third choice is to remove all reminders of the medical world; the physician is seated comfortably in front of the patient but does not wear a medical coat. None of these settings is right or wrong; they are just different. They do, however, convey different relationships between caregiver and care receiver, so room arrangement should be considered when constructing a meeting with a family to discuss bad news.

Dealing with Fear

The care provider who fears that he or she will lose his or her way during the conversation, can use the following six-step approach. The acronym *FEARED* is a mnemonic for the approach (Woods and Rozovsky, 2003).

F stands for *facts.* Describe the facts of the case in front of the family. In this way all the discussion participants hear the same thing for the first time, in its entirety.

E stands for *empathize.* When a care provider is having a discussion about an adverse outcome, it is appropriate that he or she express condolence for the outcome and be saddened that the patient must deal with such a complicated issue. This also is an opportunity for the care provider to educate by explaining certain concepts or terms that may illuminate the reasons behind the care plan.

A is for *anger.* It is important to seek sources of patient and family anger during the discussion. The provider may choose an indirect counseling style by saying: "At this stage people are in fact very angry. Do you have those feelings, and if so, where are they directed?" That question is central to the discussion, because it may be that the patient will say, "No, I don't have any angry feelings, I just feel very sad about the outcome." However, if the patient says, "Yes, I am very angry, and in fact I am angry at you," that is the opportunity for the care provider to ask the most important question, which is actually the one behind the initial question:

"How did you arrive at those conclusions?" The patient may explain issues that in fact are not understood by him or her, allowing the care provider to educate and to set the record straight. However, it is also possible that the patient in fact has an accurate assessment of the issues leading up to the adverse outcome. Under those circumstances it may be necessary for the care provider to say, "I have given your case thought every single day since it occurred, and as I look at it now, I believe if I knew the outcome when I was making those initial decisions, I might have chosen a different care plan." There are those who would suggest that this would lead to an immediate lawsuit. That is not necessarily so. On the one hand, if a patient was already going to sue, she will sue anyhow. On the other hand she may not sue simply because the care provider has offered such an honest answer.

R stands for *"please repeat back what you have heard."* We seldom as care providers ask patients to tell us what they heard. It is shocking when one gives a detailed thirty-minute discussion of an event or plan of care to find that the patient can give you only two or three components of that discussion back and cannot remember or describe the other parts of the discussion. This repeat-back technique is important because it unveils areas the patient did not understand, giving you a chance to present more information.

E is for *extended family.* It is often valuable to bring the extended family in for the initial discussion if the patient will allow that. The members of the extended family will certainly give their opinions at home, and you should know what those opinions are in order to clear up misconceptions or to understand the agenda that exists. It is possible that dynamics within the family have impaired the care that would otherwise have been given to the patient and such issues cannot come out if one does not give the extended family an opportunity to speak.

D stands for *document.* It is important to document the conversation, including the time, place, participants, topics discussed, and overall tone of the discussion. It is inappropriate to include innuendos or engage in finger pointing in such documentation because this offers nothing and in fact exposes the vulnerability of the care provider.

Conclusion

Disclosure in health care is now being viewed as an essential safety net and a foundation on which an effective care provider–patient relationship can develop. Patients who know that their care provider is being absolutely honest are much more likely to ask appropriate questions, challenge suggested therapies, and accept possibilities of adverse outcomes. Through disclosure the provider can emphasize the importance of education, address sources of anger and attitudes of family members, and monitor how well patients learn from discussions. Each of these should be done compassionately, with the care provider reaching out to the patient in a sympathetic way to enable the patient to work through the grief and anger of an adverse outcome. Once established, this form of communication is the bedrock of medicine.

References

Adams, A. M., and Smith, A. F. "Risk Perception and Communication: Recent Developments and Implications for Anesthesia." *Anaesthesia,* 2001, *56,* 745–755.

American Academy of Pediatrics, Committee on Bioethics. "Ethics and the Care of Critically Ill Infants and Children." *Pediatrics,* 1996, *98,* 149–152.

American College of Obstetricians and Gynecologists. *Code of Professional Ethics.* Washington, D.C.: American College of Obstetricians and Gynecologists, 2001.

American College of Physicians. *Ethics Manual.* (4th ed.) Washington, D.C.: American College of Physicians, 1998.

American Medical Association, Council on Ethical and Judicial Affairs. *Code of Medical Ethics: Current Opinions with Annotations.* Chicago: American Medical Association, 1997.

American Society for Healthcare Risk Management. *Perspective on Disclosure of Unanticipated Outcome Information.* Chicago: American Society for Healthcare Risk Management, June 2001.

American Society for Healthcare Risk Management. *Code of Professional Ethics and Conduct.* Chicago: American Society for Healthcare Risk Management, Sept. 2001.

American Society for Healthcare Risk Management. *Disclosure of Unanticipated Events: The Next Step in Better Communication with Patients.* Monograph: First of Three Parts. Chicago: American Society for Healthcare Risk Management, 2002.

American Society for Healthcare Risk Management. *Disclosure of Unanticipated Events: Creating an Effective Patient Communication Policy.* Monograph: Second of Three Parts. Chicago: American Society for Healthcare Risk Management, 2003.

American Society for Healthcare Risk Management. *Disclosure: What Works Now and What Can Work Even Better.* Monograph: Third of Three Parts. Chicago: American Society for Healthcare Risk Management, 2004.

Beckman, H. B., and Frankel, R. M. "The Effect of Physician Behavior on the Collection of Data." *Annals of Internal Medicine,* 1984, *101,* 692–696.

Beyth-Marom, R. "How Probable Is Probable? A Numerical Translation of Verbal Probability Expressions." *Journal of Forecasting,* 1982, *1,* 257–269.

Braddock, C. H., and others. "Informed Decision Making in an Outpatient Practice." *Journal of the American Medical Association,* 1999, *282,* 2313–2320.

Calman, K. C., and Royston, G.H.D. "Risk Language and Dialects." *British Medical Journal,* 1997, *315,* 939–942.

Coombs, R. H., Chopra, S., Schenk, D. R., and Yutan, E. "Medical Slang and Its Function." *Social Science & Medicine,* 1993, *36,* 987–998.

Elkadry, E., and others. "Do Mothers Remember Key Events During Labor?" *American Journal of Obstetrics and Gynecology,* 2003, *189,* 195–200.

Ellis, D. A., Hopkin, J. M., Leitch, A. G., and Crofton, J. "Doctors' Orders: Controlled Trial of Supplementary Written Information for Patients." *British Medical Journal,* 1979, *1,* 456.

Gallagher, T. H., and others. "Patients' and Physicians' Attitudes Regarding the Disclosure of Medical Errors." *Journal of the American Medical Association,* 2003, *289,* 1001–1007.

Gawande, A. A., and others. "Risk Factors for Retained Instruments and Sponges After Surgery." *New England Journal of Medicine*, 2003, *384*, 229–235.

Gherman, R. B. "Shoulder Dystocia: An Evidence-Based Evolution of the Obstetric Nightmare." *Clinical Obstetrics and Gynecology*, 2002, *45*, 345–362.

Grimes, D. A., and Snively, G. R. "Patients' Understanding of Medical Risks: Implications for Genetic Counseling." *Obstetrics & Gynecology*, 1999, *93*(6), 910–914.

Hickson, G. B., Clayton, E. W., Githens, P. B., and Sloan, F. A. "Factors That Prompted Families to File Medical Malpractice Following Perinatal Injuries." *Journal of the American Medical Association*, 1992, *267*, 1359–1363.

Hopper, K. D., Tenhave, T. R., Tully, D. A., and Hall, T.A.L. "The Readability of Currently Used Surgical/Procedure Consent Forms in the United States." *Surgery*, 1998, *123*, 496–503.

Joint Commission on Accreditation of Healthcare Organizations. *Comprehensive Accreditation Manual for Hospitals.* Oakbrook Terrace, Ill.: Joint Commission on Accreditation of Health Care Organizations, 2001.

Kraman, S. S., and Hamm, G. "Risk Management: Extreme Honesty May Be the Best Policy." *Annals of Internal Medicine*, 1999, *131*, 963–967.

Laudan, L. *The Book of Risks: Fascinating Facts About the Chances We Take Every Day.* New York: Wiley, 1994.

Levinson, W., Gorawara-Bhat, R., and Lamb, J. "A Study of Patient Clues and Physician Responses in Primary Care and Surgery Settings." *Journal of the American Medical Association*, 2000, *284*, 1021–1027.

Lloyd, A. J. "The Extent of Patients' Understanding of the Risk of Treatment." *Quality in Health Care*, 2001, *10*(suppl. D), i14–i18.

Lloyd, A. J., Hayes, P. D., Bell, P.R.F., and Naylor, A. R. "The Role of Risk and Benefit Perception in Informed Consent for Surgery." *Medical Decision Making*, 2001, *21*, 141–149.

Marvel, M. K., Epstein, R. M., Flowers, K., and Beckman, H. B. "Soliciting the Patients' Agenda." *Journal of the American Medical Association*, 1999, *281*, 283–287.

O'Connor, A. M., and others. "Decision Aids for Patients Facing Health Treatment or Screening Decisions: Systematic Review." *British Medical Journal*, 1999, *319*, 731–734.

Olson, J. E., and others. "Medical Record Validation of Maternally Reported Birth Characteristics and Pregnancy Related Events: A Report from the Children's Cancer Group." *American Journal of Epidemiology*, 1997, *145*, 58–67.

Rosner, F., and others. "Disclosure and Prevention of Medical Errors." *Archives of Internal Medicine*, 2000, *160*, 2089–2092.

Rozovsky, F. A. *Consent to Treatment: A Practical Guide.* (3rd ed.) Gaithersburg, Md.: Aspen, 2000 (with annual supplements through Dec. 2003).

Singh, A. D., and Paling, J. "Informed Consent: Putting Risks into Perspective." *Survey of Ophthalmology*, 1997, *42*, 83–86.

Stallings, S. P., and Paling, J. E. "New Tool for Presenting Risk in Obstetrics and Gynecology." *Obstetrics and Gynecology*, 2001, *98*, 345–349.

University of Rochester Strong Memorial Hospital. Policy 9.1.2: Disclosure of Unanticipated or Negative Outcomes. Rochester, N.Y.: University of Rochester, 2001.

Whelan, T., and others. "Mastectomy or Lumpectomy? Helping Women Make Informed Choices." *Journal of Clinical Oncology*, 1999, *17*(6), 1727–1735.

Whelan, T., and others. "Helping Patients Make Informed Choices: A Randomized Trial of a Decision Aid for Adjuvant Chemotherapy in Lymph Node-Negative Breast Cancer." *Journal of the National Cancer Institute,* 2003, *95*(8), 581–587.

Witman, A. B., Park, D. M., and Hardin, S. B. "How Do Patients Want Physicians to Handle Mistakes? A Survey of Internal Medicine Patients in an Academic Setting." *Archives of Internal Medicine,* 1996, *156,* 2565–2569.

Woods, J. R. *Describing Risks to Patients: What Do We Say? What Do They Hear?* Rochester, N.Y.: University of Rochester, Strong Perifax, 2004.

Woods, J. R., and Rozovsky, F. A. *What Do I Say? Communicating Intended or Unanticipated Outcomes in Obstetrics.* San Francisco: Jossey-Bass, 2003.

Wu, A. W. "Handling Hospital Errors: Is Disclosure the Best Defense?" *Annals of Internal Medicine,* 1999, *131,* 970–972.

CHAPTER TEN

PATIENT SAFETY IN HUMAN RESEARCH

Rodney K. Adams

Since the Second World War, autonomy and safety have been primary considerations in human research. The Nuremberg Code, The Declaration of Helsinki, and the Belmont Report are all important statements on protecting participants in human research. Similarly, federal human research regulations are focused on the informed consent and safety of research participants. The *Common Rule,* used by many federal agencies (see, for example, 45 *C.F.R.* 46, 2003), is a detailed road map of how a research protocol is to be created and implemented. Institutional review boards (IRBs) are charged with protecting research participants. Unfortunately, federal regulations do not apply to all human research in the United States and even the most detailed regulations do not preclude inadvertent lack of attention to detail. Zeal for knowledge and advancement may cloud a researcher's judgment. Therefore a health care provider engaged in research must have a consciousness of safety when drafting, implementing, and monitoring a research protocol.

Well-publicized events at many academic centers have pointed out that errors in safety are of serious concern for participants in human research. More than

This chapter is adapted from Chapter Ten of Fay A. Rozovsky and Rodney K. Adams, *Clinical Trials and Human Research: A Practical Guide to Regulatory Compliance* (San Francisco: Jossey-Bass, 2003).

a year prior to the 1999 completion of the Institute of Medicine report *To Err Is Human,* the deputy inspector general of the U.S. Department of Health and Human Services (HHS), during testimony before Congress, in essence challenged IRBs to do a better job to ensure the rights and safety of human research participants. This testimony is encapsulated in the June 1998 Office of Inspector General (OIG) report *Institutional Review Boards: A Time for Reform* (Department of Health and Human Services, OIG, 1998). The OIG called for *data safety monitoring boards* (DSMBs) that would provide summary assessments of adverse event reports to IRBs so that the IRBs could better assess the ongoing safety of research trials. Further, the OIG recommended elimination of the *forum shopping* done when sponsors unhappy with the reviews carried out by one IRB take their protocols to another IRB without telling the second board about the earlier one's involvement or determinations. The OIG viewed this as denying the second IRB important information and short-circuiting the opportunity for human subject protection. In keeping with the theme of human subject protection, the OIG recommended that IRBs become more involved with what transpires during research trials. For particularly high-risk trials, this might involve the use of intermediaries, counselors, or other third parties to observe the consent process. IRB members might conduct random unannounced visits to review relevant documentation and to oversee the consent process.

The OIG reported in April 2000 that a number of changes had been made in human research programs but that many recommendations remained unheeded (HHS, OIG, 2000). Some of these recommendations involved patient safety. During this time frame, major structural changes in federal oversight were initiated involving the Office for Protection from Research Risks (OPRR), a part of the National Institutes of Health (NIH) with authority over NIH-funded research. In June 2000, the secretary of Health and Human Services replaced OPRR with the Office for Human Research Protections (OHRP), which reports directly to the secretary. Positioned at the departmental level, the new agency was designed to provide "leadership" for the federal agencies funding human research. Since its inception OHRP has moved to develop strategies for educating IRB members and clinical investigators and to improve regulatory compliance.

This chapter describes a practical approach to enhancing the safety of human research as well as to responding to adverse events. The work of DSMBs is examined. Research strategies that lessen the risk of adverse events and unanticipated outcomes are also described. Management of concurrent situations, incident reporting, and sentinel event reporting are discussed in the context of human research.

Creating a Patient Safety Environment for Clinical Trials

A number of practical steps can be implemented to create a safer environment for human research. These steps include employing effective screening tools to identify participants who are at risk of experiencing an adverse event, having appropriate consent procedures, having an effective on-call system, using signage and checklists, supplying participants with MedicAlert-style bracelets, and educating all involved. Making vital information available to a participant's other health care providers as well as responding to a participant's concerns in a timely manner is important. A related concept is having a contingency plan for adverse events. Each of these categories is discussed in the following sections.

Screening Tools

Critical to successful management of a clinical trial is the proper selection of research participants. The participants must meet the study design requirements; however, they may also present with a constellation of risk factors. These risk factors may have nothing to do with the clinical study, yet in some cases their presence should bar the individual from inclusion in the investigation. For example, a trial might involve investigation of a new diabetes medication. Screening information obtained from an individual may clearly indicate that he or she is eligible for the study. However, additional scrutiny may reveal a history of noncompliance with structured medication schedules. No familial caregiver or friend who might assist the individual with staying on the required regimen is available. Because it is critical for participants to stay within the rigid parameters of the study, this is a person *at risk,* who probably should not be enrolled in the study.

Consent Tools

Consent is a pivotal component in human research and clinical trials. It is equally important for a participant's safety. Consent is more than securing a written authorization for inclusion in a study; it is a communication tool that enables the principal investigator and study personnel to impart important information for safe participation in a research protocol. Disclosure of possible anticipated side effects should always be part of the discussion. However, from a safety perspective, what is equally important is to use the consent process as a forum for schooling participants on what steps to take if such side effects occur. Additionally, research consent procedures usually include some discussion about "unforeseeable" risk factors. Participants may have unusual or unanticipated responses to a study intervention or an investigational drug. Rather than having these responses dismissed as "nothing to worry about," participants should be encouraged to report them promptly. A practice that is gaining more acceptance is to involve a family member of the participant in the consent process. This can be done only with the permission of the research participant. The rationale is that the family member may have a perspective different from the participant's on key issues such as predisposing risk factors, ability to adhere to the protocol, and early detection of adverse events. At the same time, the family member can school others about what to look for in terms of reactions or adverse events and the appropriate response to such situations. For example, a participant may be enrolled in a study that involves an implanted investigational cardiac pacemaker device. He collapses at home on the living room floor, and 911 is called. The emergency medical services response team has no idea that the individual is enrolled in a clinical trial. No one in the immediate family is aware of the individual's role in the study, and so they are unable to shed light on what might have caused the person to collapse. The unfortunate result is a therapeutic intervention that is incompatible with the study, resulting in harm to the subject-patient. The chance of avoiding such real-life risk situations is increased if one or more family members are involved from the outset in the communication process called *consent*. As a communication tool the consent process can be used to reinforce the importance of alerting study personnel to risk-prone situations and aid those assisting a subject-patient who requires a therapeutic intervention.

Checklists

A practical approach to maintaining research participant safety involves the use of checklists. When used as guidelines or pathways, these tools are not "cookbook" clinical research. Instead, they serve as reminders or helpful algorithms for reducing unwanted or risk-prone variations in the proper management of a clinical protocol. Some of the checklists can be for the use of clinical research staff. Others can be useful guides for inpatient, emergency department, and urgent care personnel who encounter research participants as patients. Finally, yet other checklists can provide important reminders to research participants and their family members about what to do when reactions or adverse effects occur.

On-Call Systems and Interactive Web Sites

Other measures are also important in maintaining excellent communication. One involves having an effective on-call protocol so that when research participants call with questions or to report what they believe is an adverse event, someone can respond quickly. This is especially important in high-risk trials and also in those protocols in which the consent document "assures" participants that if they call, *someone will get back to them promptly.* An on-call system may forward calls to someone carrying a cell phone or a pager. In practical terms this means there *must be timely follow-through* in returning calls. Another technique is to provide participants with the Internet address for a secure Web site. (This presupposes that research participants have access to the Internet.) Using their protocol identification number or a similar code process, research participants could visit a Web site that includes frequently asked questions (FAQs) and answers to common concerns stemming from involvement in the research trial. It might also have a monitored chat room or "e-mail us" function through which participants could receive prompt answers to such questions as, "Am I experiencing an adverse reaction to the study drug?" or, "I missed two of my medications yesterday and this morning. What should I do?" For the Web site approach to meet participants' needs, someone on the study staff must *monitor* the Web and e-mail traffic and ensure that a timely response is made. (Some investigators have complained that research participants are organizing their own chat rooms and causing problems such as unblinding studies. This may lead to the participants' reaching incorrect conclusions about the study drug or to the participants' being influenced by the group discussion. An official Web site that addresses the primary concerns of the participants with reliable responses is a better course.) The Internet provides a powerful tool for overseeing the participants' concerns and questions and for averting possible harm to participants and reducing the likelihood that they will drop out of the investigation. In this way Web site information might contribute to enhancements in the study design.

Signage

Signage is also an important step toward creating a culture of safety for clinical research trials. It involves well-displayed notices in languages used by members of the community in which the facility is situated. Signage is particularly important in hospitals, freestanding urgent care units, ambulatory patient care units, and retail pharmacies. The message to be communicated is simple:

> Are You Taking Part in a Clinical Trial or Research?
> If so, please tell us when you register for treatment.

These signs are a friendly reminder, a prompt to disclose an important consideration that caregivers need to take into account when evaluating a patient's needs, performing therapeutic interventions, or prescribing medication. Why place the same type of signage at multiple locations? The rationale is simple: these messages are a communication safety net to catch research participants who might otherwise miss an opportunity to provide salient information about participation in a clinical trial that has or could have an adverse impact on proposed treatment. For example, a research subject-patient might have missed the prompt at the free-standing urgent care center she visited. However, seeing it at the retail pharmacy she visits next, the participant says to the pharmacy technician, "Yes, I am in a study. Why is that important? After all, the doctor only prescribed some antibiotics and over-the-counter pain medication." It is important because this may be the last opportunity to prevent an untoward synergistic effect between an investigational drug and routine medical treatment. When told about her participation in the study, the pharmacy technician should inform the pharmacist. In turn the pharmacist should contact the prescribing doctor, who should discuss the treatment with a study investigator or coordinator. This conversation may turn out to be an early warning of an adverse effect or it may be about a routine infection that has nothing to do with the study. At the very least the communication provides peace of mind for the patient, prescribing physician, and investigator and allows a decision to be made about the next steps, such as clearing the proposed prescription or suggesting an alternative. The root of this safety process is the signage in the retail pharmacy that prompted the research participant to notify staff about her involvement in a research protocol.

Research Bracelets

Many individuals wear bracelets or necklaces emblazoned with medical warnings or alerts. Some include information about allergies, underlying medical conditions, medication requirements, or organ donor status. Still others provide instructions on resuscitation requests. The information is designed to alert first responders and emergency department personnel about what to do when assisting the person wearing the bracelet or necklace. It is a very practical idea for clinical trial participants and can increase their safety. Study participants often travel miles away from the location in which they participate in an investigation. If a participant then requires medical attention, there is no way in which his caregivers would know that he was enrolled in a study unless he were to tell them. He might need treatment as the result of an adverse reaction to a study drug or injuries sustained in an unrelated event. Without the benefit of knowing that the patient is taking part in a research protocol, care providers may make a misdiagnosis or provide inappropriate treatment given the medications or devices involved in the clinical study. Providing participants with warning bracelets or necklaces can greatly reduce this risk to participant safety. Bracelet or necklace information should include the following:

- The name of the *protocol*
- The patient's clinical research *identification number*
- A *toll-free number or e-mail address* to contact for urgent information

In addition the information should include a warning statement, as follows:

Warning!
I am enrolled in a clinical research study. Please contact the
study coordinator before performing treatment!

Taking this additional step helps to ensure the safety of research participants. It also may help to maintain the integrity of the study, so that participants are not lost to follow-up as a result of an unfortunate response to a need for treatment.

Even though individually identifiable information is involved, it is possible to create a HIPAA (Health Insurance Portability and Accountability Act) compliant, firewall-protected Web site for posting important clinical trial information needed for the treatment of a research participant who takes ill miles away from the clinical trial location. A secure Web site that is password protected is much more useful to a treating physician than are records locked in a file cabinet at night. The information is available to a treating physician regardless of where in the world the research participant might travel. Tracking access to the Web site is no more difficult than for any electronic medical record.

Education

Everyone involved in clinical research trials can benefit from safety education. Providing staff with practical training on safety practices can prevent them and the participants from experiencing harm. The same is true for research participants and their families: understanding the protocol, knowing what to look for in terms of early warning signs of adverse effects, and knowing how to interact with the research staff and treatment facilities can all contribute to positive outcomes. Offering such education provides a useful way of addressing issues that may become life- or health-threatening events, and it may improve the quality of clinical data. Rather than letting situations evolve into crises, the prudent approach is to anticipate possible adverse events through cogent education that leads to successful strategies for avoiding or managing problems.

These measures are illustrative of the steps to take to create a culture of safety in studies that use human participants. Other steps may be added that are consistent with ongoing patient safety strategies in a health care organization or a contract research organization.

Continuous Quality Assurance

Vitally important in all aspects of health care, continuous quality assurance is equally important in human research. It may take the shape of random auditing, skills checklists, participant interviews, and other tools that can ensure that the research protocol is being followed. A certain amount of redundancy, in the form of double-checks, increases in importance as the risk of harm to a participant increases in a study. When the line between a medication's therapeutic dosage and fatal dosage is very small, who draws up the drug, how and where the drug is administered, and how the event is documented are all part of the quality assurance process.

Responding to Adverse Events

The first and foremost objective in health care is to provide care to the patient. This is equally true when responding to a potentially adverse event in a research protocol. Treatment of the patient is the first priority. Then comes the paperwork. It is imperative that IRBs receive prompt notification about adverse events stemming from research studies. These events include situations in which participants experience serious harm or unforeseen accidents or problems. When an adverse event such as a serious injury or a death occurs, a thorough review is warranted. A failure analysis or root cause analysis is warranted to ascertain why the event occurred. The results may be surprising.

Clinical Contingency Plan for Adverse Events

Along with properly trained personnel to field questions and the use of warning bracelets or necklaces, a plan should be in place to manage the care of participants who experience an adverse event. Such a plan should include

- *Having clinical management algorithms* for differentiating adverse reactions to a device or drug under investigation in the study and the results of drug-drug or drug-food interactions or other factors
- *Having a procedure for notifying the clinical care team* about study-related adverse events and successful treatment plans from other episodes when the adverse events occurred.

- *Providing instruction sheets to participants* at the time of their enrollment in the study reminding them to alert their primary care provider, family, and urgent care or emergency department staff that they are involved in a clinical trial of an investigational drug or device
- *Providing instruction sheets to on-call personnel and those monitoring e-mail traffic* on how to manage the situation when a participant is believed to be experiencing an adverse event
- *Following-up* once care is completed to determine what worked and what did not work in managing the condition suffered by the participant who has experienced an adverse event related to the drug or device under investigation

Analysis of Adverse Events

Although many observers may be ready to ascribe the adverse event that causes injury or death to the investigational device or drug, it may instead prove to be the culmination of a series of system failures. Delving into the issue is worthwhile as it could mean correcting system failures rather than suspending a valid research protocol. Models exist for this type of investigation, including those with which accredited hospitals are familiar (such as the Framework for Conducting a Root Cause Analysis, available from the Joint Commission on Accreditation of Healthcare Organizations [JCAHO]) and those with which many manufacturing industries are conversant (such as PROACT, root cause failure analysis software from the Reliability Center). It must be appreciated, however, that even if a timely and thorough investigation of an adverse event occurs, it may not preclude the possibility of litigation stemming from an injury to or the death of a participant, investigation by a coroner or medical examiner, criminal probes by law enforcement, or compliance oversight investigations by pertinent federal or state regulatory bodies such as the Food and Drug Administration (FDA), the Office for Human Research Protections (OHRP), or a state Board of Medicine.

A Systematic Approach to Managing Adverse Events

With such an array of possible regulatory investigations, it is important that health care facilities or contract research organizations have in place a systematic approach to investigating, managing, and promptly reporting the findings on adverse events. Such an approach would include the following considerations:

Investigation. Once an adverse event occurs an investigation should be started immediately to determine what gave rise to it. Care should be taken not to jump to conclusions but rather to look at processes that should have occurred and to compare this information with what is learned about what did occur. For example, a research participant may have received ten times the dose of radiation expected in the research protocol. The investigators should not jump to the conclusion that "somebody did something wrong." Rather, they should look at documentation, communication, and equipment calibration processes as well as staff education. Taking this approach it may turn out that several processes or procedures failed and coalesced into a systems failure. Alternatively, human factors may be involved. It may be found that a staffer "took it for granted" that the radiation machine was always set at the proper parameters and did not bother to double-check the calibrations per study protocol. In this situation the adverse event involves a human failure as well as a systems failure, implicating a lack of fail-safes to prevent such an adverse event.

Sequestration of Documentation. As part of an investigation all pertinent documentation should be obtained and copies sequestered pending the disposition of the matter. This does not mean, however, that the original documents must be sequestered. Rather, verified copies can be maintained for investigative purposes. The copies should be date and time stamped to indicate when they were prepared, along with the name and position of the person doing the copying. Most qualified health information specialists are conversant with applicable state laws that address the "usual and customary" business practices that may be used to prepare a credible, authenticated copy of such records. Taking these measures does not impede the use of the original record for purposes of ongoing research work or the treatment of the research participant.

Sequestration of Ancillary Record Information. Paper documentation alone is not sufficient for purposes of an adverse event investigation. As with hard copy information, verified copies should be made of electronic record data. These copies should be preserved in a format that is timed and dated and impervious to modification. This format should also include the name and title of the individual who makes the reproduction. A recognized process should be used so that the reproduction will be considered authentic.

Sequestration of Equipment. It is important to secure any devices involved in an adverse event, including investigational devices. Care should be taken in the handling of such equipment too. Specific procedures should be in place that address who may examine the device and whether the equipment may be removed from the premises for this purpose. Manufacturers' warranty language often carries warnings that any tampering with or removal of the factory seal on a device breaches the warranty. However, when the manufacturer's representative and a biomedical engineer from a reputable third party examine the device, this does not void the warranty. The idea of a third party viewing a medical device can prove very sensitive. A confidentiality agreement may be necessary to allay fears that intellectual property may be stolen. Then, although the representative from the third-party biomedical engineering firm may examine the device and document or testify about the findings, he or she will be precluded by the confidentiality agreement from sharing or using the information for any other purpose.

Interviews. An important part of the adverse event investigation is to get information from firsthand observers. The interviews to accomplish this should be carefully constructed to avoid biases or presuppositions about what transpired. All those involved in the event, from those who prepared the protocol, test article, or equipment to the person carrying out the protocol should be interviewed. Interviews with the study participant are equally important. Documentation for the interviews should include the following:

- The subject (topic) of the interview
- The interviewer's name and title
- The interview time, date, and location
- A list of the questions posed
- The responses to the questions

    The assistance of an attorney will be needed to determine whether these interviews can be considered privileged and thus protected from disclosure and what steps will be necessary to ensure that the privilege is applicable.

Process Indicators. An adverse event investigation can be time consuming and expensive. Because the results may mean suspension of a trial or a regulatory sanction, it is important to take a consistent, meticulous approach to examining adverse events. A series of *process indicators,* or *prompts,* can be used to guarantee a consistent and thorough approach to adverse event investigations:

Identify Processes Involved in the Event

- Consent
- Confidentiality
- Medication
- Surgery
- Radiation
- Chemotherapy
- Physical therapy

- Psychotherapy
- Behavior management or modification
- Investigational device
- Investigational drug
- Combination investigational device and conventional treatment (describe treatment)
- Combination investigational drug and conventional treatment (describe treatment)
- Clinical trial staff education and training
- Education and training for research participants and family members
- Identification of onset of adverse event
- Communication linked to identification of onset of adverse event
- Reporting of adverse event
- Treatment for adverse event

Answer These Questions

- Have authenticated copies of relevant documentation been obtained?
- Have authenticated copies of electronic files been obtained?
- Has equipment been sequestered?
- Have interviews been completed? For each interview supply
  Name
  Title (if applicable)
  Date of interview
  Interviewer

For Each Process Identified, Answer These Questions

- Did a process variance occur?
- If yes, describe the variance.

List Identified Opportunities for Process Improvement

A Visual Algorithm for Adverse Event Investigations. Those who must manage an adverse event may find it very useful to construct a flowchart. It should depict the steps to take in identifying, managing, and reporting an adverse event in a research protocol.

Communication About an Adverse Event

Communicating about an adverse event involves determining what reports are needed, to whom the reports should be made, and how study participants will be involved. In most cases, an adverse event will need to be reported to several entities in a very short time period.

Determining Whether the Event Requires Reporting. One important aspect of the investigation is determining what types of reports must be completed subsequent to an adverse event. The threshold consideration, however, is determining whether an individual's outcome constitutes an adverse event. The definition of *adverse event* may vary among interested constituencies. For example, an end-user, device-related serious injury may trigger reporting under the Safe Medical Devices Act and its accompanying regulations. If an individual is receiving both accepted treatment (patient) and an experimental protocol (research participant), there may be no obligation to report the situation to the IRB. In practical terms, however, it may be prudent to notify the IRB even when a nonresearch aspect of the participant's treatment leads to an adverse outcome. Moreover, even if federal regulations do not trigger a reporting obligation in such situations, a contract with a private sponsor may do so. For example, the sponsor of an experimental drug under investigation for treatment of cancer might want to know that the serious injury to a study participant came about *not* as a result of the study but for totally different reasons. The point is that an investigation should yield sufficient information with which to make a reporting determination. Unfortunately, the time limit within which a report must be made often gives investigators little opportunity to determine the cause of the adverse event.

Determining Who Must Receive a Report. When an adverse event occurs, it may trigger reporting obligations under any of several federal, state, and contractual requirements. A number of questions should be asked in determining report recipients:

- Did the adverse event stem from a clinical protocol, or was the individual a participant in a clinical trial *and* a patient receiving accepted treatment?
- Did the adverse event involve an approved or an investigational device?
- Did the adverse event involve an approved drug or a drug under investigation?
- Did the adverse event involve an approved drug that was being tested for a new use?
- Did the adverse event result in the unexpected death of the participant?
- Did the adverse event occur in a JCAHO-accredited facility? If so, did it constitute a *reviewable event* as defined by JCAHO?
- Has the adverse event triggered a mandatory reporting obligation under applicable state law?
- Does the adverse event require a report to the sponsor under the terms of the agreement with the sponsor?

- Does the adverse event require a report to the IRB under the policies and procedures of the IRB?
- Does the adverse event require a report to other facilities carrying out the same or similar studies, under the terms of the protocol, the policies and procedures of the IRB, or the agreement with the sponsor?
- Does the adverse event require the notification of either the quality assurance or risk management officer under the policies and procedures of the health care facility or contract research organization?
- If the facility in which the adverse event took place is obliged to follow the Conditions of Participation in Medicare or Medicaid for hospitals, is there a requirement to notify senior management of participant complaints or grievances linked to a research-related adverse event?
- If the health care organization has a corporate compliance plan, is there a responsibility to notify the compliance officer about a research-related adverse event?
- Is there a responsibility to notify liability insurance carriers about a research-related adverse event? If the health care organization has an insurance captive, is there an obligation to report to the captive manager?
- If the adverse event is related to competency, misrepresentation, fraud, deceit, or unprofessional conduct, is there an obligation to report to state licensing bodies or the federal Office of Research Integrity?

Depending on the circumstances of the specific case, the answers to these questions may identify *multiple* reporting obligations. Some of these reporting obligations may compete with or conflict with one another in terms of order of priority and the amount of detail to be provided in each instance.

To be certain that all the necessary reports are made, it is suggested that the IRB and research office personnel work together to develop a *reporting matrix*. Developed by a team of key stakeholders, this chart can summarize all the necessary tracking information: when reports should be made, to whom, and in what priority. Any concerns about adverse event reporting should be referred to the risk management department or legal counsel. The multidisciplinary approach is important for capturing all the information about the need to report. Thus the design team may include representatives from the IRB, legal counsel, and research office and from the compliance, risk management, and accreditation functions of the health care organization. When state and federal laws respecting reporting are changed, the reporting matrix should be updated accordingly. To be certain that adverse events do not go unreported, the matrix should be provided to principal investigators and their key administrative staff. Protocol approval should be contingent upon meeting the IRB's policy on adverse event reporting. Training on the importance of reporting should also be included in the staff education process.

Managing Multiple Reporting Obligations. There is always the chance that one adverse event report may appear to contradict another report about the same adverse event. What investigators and others involved in preparing reports must focus on, however, is the information required for meeting the reporting obligations set by each report recipient. For example, a sponsor's agreement may oblige the principal investigator to report the deaths of all study participants. It may, however, go on to specify, "Please provide a detailed report only if the participant's death was known to be or believed to be related to the investigational device." Therefore, if the investigator found that a medication was involved in the participant's demise, the sponsor would not receive a detailed report on that cause. At the same time, detailed information may be part of a root cause analysis completed by the JCAHO-accredited hospital in which the person was a participant in the research trial. On their face, the reports might appear contradictory. However, each report is made for a specific *purpose,* and in each instance the information supplied meets the reporting requirements.

Difficulties do arise when those required to receive essentially the same information end up with contradictory reports. This is not acceptable, and all reports should be reviewed carefully to be certain that the information is accurate and complete for the recipient's purpose. Inconsistencies should trigger a further review of the draft reports.

Federal regulations set out a process for addressing adverse events affecting human research participants. The Common Rule (for example, 45 *C.F.R.* 46, 2003) is used by most federal agencies that fund or oversee human research. The FDA has a separate set of regulations (21 *C.F.R.* 312, 2003) that are similar but not identical to the common rule for investigating the efficacy and safety of new drugs and devices. For example, under the Common Rule, an IRB must have a written process in place for prompt reporting by an investigator of unanticipated problems involving risks to research participants. Under FDA *investigational new drug* (IND) requirements the sponsor of the IND has to notify the FDA and participating investigators, in a written safety report, of any adverse experience associated with the use of the drug that is both serious and unexpected. The FDA also may request that the sponsor telephone or fax reports of unexpected fatal or life-threatening experiences associated with the use of the drug as soon as possible. The requirement must be met no later than seven calendar days after the day that the sponsor received the information. This means that the IRB and clinical investigators must be cognizant of the different reporting triggers for research conducted under HHS regulations and that conducted under the FDA's IND protocols.

Under the Conditions of Participation in Medicare and Medicaid for hospitals, a patient is entitled to file a grievance under the patient's rights standards. This will trigger a detailed probe and report. It may be quite a challenge to sort out the conventional treatment-related events from those that took place under the aegis of the clinical research protocol in which the individual is enrolled. This multiplicity of investigations and fact finding, all done in the name of creating a safe environment, could prove expensive and time consuming and may generate contradictory results owing to the differences in the regulations. Final analysis may generate a confirmation that the patient has a genuine point of grievance, but on the research side there may be no basis for considering the occurrence an adverse event.

From the point of view of accreditors, an event may constitute an *unanticipated outcome,* triggering yet a different type of reporting to the patient, as described in the patient safety standards published by the Joint Commission on Accreditation of Healthcare Organizations. This is an important consideration when trying to put in place the infrastructure for a patient-subject safety-oriented protocol.

A health care provider is constantly challenged to determine when an adverse event has actually occurred and to make timely reports to the appropriate entities. Failure to fulfill reporting obligations can be embarrassing and very costly in many ways.

Disclosing Information to Research Participants. Study participants should be told when it is determined that they have experienced a research-related adverse event. This report is part of the ongoing communication that is so important in restoring public confidence in the safety of human research programs. That an adverse event has occurred *does not* mean, however, that there must be an admission of liability or culpability. In fact the disclosure may be made before an investigation determines the cause or causes of the adverse event. What participants want to know is quite understandable:

- What does this mean to me?
- Will I recover?
- How long will my recovery take?
- Does this episode mean I am out of the study?
- Who pays for my continued care?
- I want to complain about what happened. Whom do I contact?

A related issue is what should be disclosed to the participant's family or the legally authorized representative. If the participant has authorized the involvement of family members or surrogates, there should be no difficulty in disclosing information about the adverse event. However, if a participant has specifically asked that information not be revealed to family members or a legally authorized representative, that request should be respected. Some exceptions may be permitted under the terms of state law or the HIPAA regulations dealing with health information.

What may be more problematic for some investigators is revealing to unaffected research participants that other participants have experienced adverse events. Some argue that by disclosing this information, investigators could bias the study by planting the suggestion that the currently unaffected participant might experience similar adverse events. Others argue that it is important to be open and honest with participants and to let them know when adverse events have become a documented part of the study. (Some argue that this is required as part of the ongoing informed consent process.) In between these viewpoints is a third perspective. This middle stance looks to the facts and circumstances of the adverse event. If it is one that is likely to be experienced throughout the study population, it is information that participants should receive so that they can pinpoint the event if they experience it and take appropriate action. However, if it is a rare event, the IRB may not require the investigator to disclose this finding if doing so may jeopardize the integrity of the study or prevent the research from going forward or if the risk of harm to other participants is minimal. At the very least, once the adverse event is known to occur the IRB and sponsor should be notified so that an ethical and legal decision can be made about disseminating information to the study population.

Giving Participants Directions for Adverse Event Reporting. Research participants need clear, understandable information about what is considered an adverse event. Some reactions may be anticipated whereas others may not. To be certain that participants understand what an adverse event is and what they should do when such an event occurs, it is prudent for research coordinators to do the following:

- Develop standard information to be provided to all research participants.
- Test the comprehensibility of this information by using it with a sample of individuals who may become research participants and those who may act as their legally authorized representatives.
- Adjust the language to meet the reading level of the potential study population.
- Develop in-service training for investigators and their staff that gives them practical ways to teach participants to identify and report adverse events.
- Obtain input from and the approval of the IRB for the standard information format.

Educating Participants About Emergency Treatment for Adverse Events. Because many research studies are based in hospitals or near such facilities, participants are often encouraged to seek assistance at the hospital emergency
department. Some research consent documents or instruction sheets state, "Should
you experience a problem and you are unable to contact us, please proceed to our
[or a named] emergency department and they will be able to assist you." This type
of language often alarms health care attorneys and risk managers as it creates the
impression that there is a legal relationship between the study and the hospital
emergency department. Moreover, such instructions, implying that the emergency
department is informed about the study and its participants, are seen as creating
a false sense of security. The emergency department personnel may not have any
idea that the individual is enrolled in a study. Even when that information is
known, they may not know what treatment the study involves and if in fact it re-
lates to the presenting ailment. A related concern is the notation on some instruction sheets that directs participants to "call or e-mail our office night or day
if you have an adverse event or problem." Unless the phone line or e-mail system
is monitored around the clock, a research participant could wait hours for a response. What might have been a manageable adverse event at the outset may
become impossible to control over that time. In addition, giving participants the
expectation that they have access to a constantly monitored phone line or e-mail
system when they do not could constitute a liability risk exposure.

Researchers can explore several practical options for avoiding needless delay
in responding to an adverse event. For example:

- Provide a phone *rollover* service; calls that are not picked up after five or six rings
  are forwarded to a staffed call center.
- Make certain the call center can always reach a research staff member who can
  respond to the participant within a defined time period.
- Make certain the pager system is staffed twenty-four hours a day.
- Have the e-mail message system linked to a pager, cell phone, or personal
  digital assistant (PDA) to alert the on-call research staff member to respond
  to the participant.
- Perform quality audits to be certain that voice and e-mail messages are
  answered within a designated time period.

If a decision is made to encourage participants to seek emergency services
at a designated facility or to telephone an on-call medical group, it is important
that the facility or group have sufficient background information on the study to
plan appropriate treatment. As was suggested earlier, this is why there is merit in
providing participants with a MedicAlert-style bracelet or necklace. With pertinent

information such as the study number, participant identifier, and a staffed toll-free number to call or Internet Web address to contact, the MedicAlert-style notification gives caregivers a way to access important details needed in treating a participant who presents with an adverse event.

Using Data and Safety Monitoring Boards

When constructing a research protocol, an investigator must ensure that ongoing evaluation of study data occurs as these data are accumulated. In an FDA-regulated study, data monitoring is also the responsibility of the sponsor. An IRB must ensure that this critical element is part of a research protocol. Using an independent group, often called a *data and safety monitoring board* (DSMB), to perform this function is an excellent way to achieve objective analysis of study information, says the Office for Human Research Protections (HHS, OHRP, 2002). (DSMBs are occasionally referred to as *data monitoring committees* [DMCs], particularly in FDA publications.)

A DSMB can analyze interim data, often from multiple sites, as well as external data from other studies and reports. A DSMB should be evaluating the efficacy of the therapy under study, its relative merit compared to other treatments (including no treatment), and any adverse events causally related to the therapy. Often the DSMB is the first to be in a position to make a sound judgment that a study should be terminated because the investigational therapy is clearly superior or inferior to the control therapy or patient safety is clearly in jeopardy. More often, a DSMB will recommend that a study continue, as a conclusion cannot yet be supported statistically. A DSMB may also recommend alterations to the protocol, the populations enrolled, or the information that should be supplied to participants.

The OIG believes that an IRB alone cannot provide a sufficient degree of protection to research participants and that DSMBs can play a vital role when trials pose significant risks to patients (HHS, OIG, 2000, p. 4). The OIG has recommended that DSMBs be required for certain high-risk and multisite trials, believing that "DSMBs are independent assessment bodies that provide medical, scientific and other expertise that is not typically available on IRBs, thereby serving an invaluable function in protecting human subjects" (HHS, OIG, 2000, p. 12). However, an IRB does not absolve itself of responsibility for protecting research participants when it employs a DSMB. A DSMB is merely a useful tool for an IRB to use in fulfilling its responsibility. A DSMB should provide summary assessments of a study's adverse event reports to the overseeing IRB(s). "IRBs are swamped with individual adverse event reports from multi-site trials, but these reports lack the essential context to confer meaning about the relative safety of the trial. DSMBs can provide this context and thereby enhance the IRB's capacity to assess the ongoing safety of a trial" (HHS, OIG, 2000, p. 12). In addition, a DSMB decides how missing or suspect data are to be handled in overall analyses of a study.

Indications for Use

DSMBs have gained favor in large, randomized, multisite studies that evaluate interventions intended to prolong life or reduce the risk of a major adverse health outcome such as a cardiac event or recurrence of cancer (FDA, 2001). They are generally not practical in short-term studies where a DSMB would not have the opportunity to analyze the data in a timely fashion. The FDA has suggested that the following criteria should be considered when determining whether to employ a DSMB:

1. Risk to study participants
2. Practicality of DSMB review
3. Assurance of scientific validity

A study sponsor, especially in sponsor-designed pharmaceutical and medical device studies, often considers whether use of a DSMB is indicated. A DSMB can help a sponsor meet its obligation to monitor studies evaluating new drugs, biologics, and devices and report adverse events to the FDA (21 *C.F.R.* §§ 312.50 and 312.56, 2003, for drugs and biologics; 21 *C.F.R.* §§ 812.40 and 812.46, 2003, for devices). Many sponsors now routinely use a DSMB as part of clinical trials. Prudence would counsel use of a DSMB in any study where the ability to monitor data is beyond the resources of the local IRB. However, FDA regulations do not require the use of a DSMB, except for studies in emergency settings (under 21 *C.F.R.* § 50.24[a][7][iv], 2003) where informed consent may be waived.

An IRB should determine at the time of its initial assessment whether a DSMB is required. What is the complexity of the study? Is mortality or major morbidity a primary or secondary end point? What is the size and duration of the study? What is the degree of risk? Are the subjects members of a fragile population, such as children or the elderly? A DSMB is intended to review unblinded interim data. An IRB can rely on the recommendations of a DSMB. A DSMB usually does not monitor a single test site for protocol compliance or appropriate data entry.

The NIH (1998) gives excellent guidance on the use of DSMBs in NIH-funded or NIH-conducted trials. Phase 3 trials generally are required to have DSMBs, and most DSMB engagements involve site monitoring as part of the quality assurance program of the funding institute or center. The NIH (2000) also recommends the use of a DSMB or similar arrangement for certain Phase 1 and Phase 2 studies, especially when large numbers of participants are enrolled or multiple sites are used. DSMBs associated with NIH trials are expected to forward summary reports of adverse events to IRBs (NIH, 1999).

Composition

Unfortunately, federal regulations and policy statements give little guidance about the quantity of individuals who should serve on a DSMB or about those individuals' attributes. The FDA (2001) has noted that a DSMB may have as few as three members, but it encourages a broader group than this. Ideally, some members will have scientific backgrounds useful in evaluating the data being collected from an investigation. A biostatistician needs to undertake the analysis of the data. Whether the biostatistician should be a member of the DSMB is debated. Specialists in pharmacokinetics, toxicology, epidemiology, and the medical specialty of the study may be needed. The FDA (2001) has also suggested that adequate representation of gender, ethnicity, and the disease process under study is important. Equally important are the independence and the influence of the DSMB. Thus the members must have standing in the scientific community sufficient to make them effective in persuading an investigator, an IRB, and the sponsor to modify or terminate a study when that course is indicated by data analysis.

Some sponsors create DSMBs from their own upper scientific management teams. Such a DSMB has the benefits of being organized easily, efficient in gathering the members for a meeting, and usually persuasive in its recommendations. However, it may suffer from being pressured explicitly or implicitly to minimize the significance of adverse events or to accept dubious clinical data as showing the effectiveness of the investigational drug. The FDA (2001) points out that sponsors may feel pressured to make a premature disclosure of results because of SEC reporting requirements, fiduciary responsibilities, and other business considerations and that an independent DSMB protects the sponsor from such poor decisions. Thus a better approach than the DSMB made up entirely of members of internal scientific management is a DSMB with a sufficient number of independent members to ensure that data are analyzed critically and appropriate responses are made. Clearly, a study investigator or participant should not be a member of the study's DSMB. Scientists who have outspoken views on the merits of the therapy under investigation should also not be on the DSMB.

Relationship to an IRB

A DSMB will collect and interpret data from all of a study's clinical sites. Often each IRB will approve and give continued approval to only one research site.

Therefore the DSMB may be able to spot significant data earlier by seeing data from more than one location and from a larger population. "IRBs conducting continuing review of research may rely on a current statement from the DSMB indicating that it has evaluated study-wide adverse events, interim findings, and any recent literature that may be relevant to the research, in lieu of requiring that this information be submitted directly to the IRB. Of course, the IRB still must receive and review reports of local, on-site unanticipated problems involving risks to participants or others and any other information needed to ensure that its continuing review is substantive and meaningful" (HHS, OHRP, 2002). The IRB always maintains the responsibility of protecting patients at its site. Although it may rely on reports from the DSMB, it has the responsibility of taking whatever actions are necessary to protect the participants.

Activities

The activities of a DSMB should be structured like those of an IRB. Participant safety, public relations, and scientific validity require that the DSMB operate in a logical and predictable manner. Policies and procedures should be written and followed. These should include a schedule of meetings and the format for each meeting, the format for presenting data to the DSMB, the format for reporting interim findings, and the statistical methods to be used. Minutes of every meeting should be written in detail and filed. The board's recommendations should be communicated clearly to the sponsor. A DSMB usually does not report directly to the FDA unless its doing so is part of the study's design. However, the sponsor has an obligation to report the DSMB's recommendations in a timely manner to the FDA and the responsible IRB(s). The DSMB's activities are reviewed as part of the FDA's consideration of the study data.

The NIH Model for Data and Safety Monitoring

As mentioned previously, the National Institutes of Health require data and safety monitoring, generally through a DSMB, for Phase 3 clinical trials sponsored by NIH. It also recommends a DSMB for Phase 1 and Phase 2 clinical trials when these studies (1) have multiple clinical sites, (2) are blind (masked), or (3) employ particularly high-risk interventions or vulnerable populations. Conversely, an independent DSMB may not be necessary or appropriate when the proposed intervention is low risk. Monitoring by the investigator or by an independent individual may be sufficient. When a DSMB is employed, an IRB can rely on the summary reports of adverse events from the DSMB (NIH, 2000).

Conclusion

Research participant safety will remain a core issue for regulators and participants. Steps can be taken to minimize needless risk exposure for research participants. Communicating with all involved in a study, documenting activities, training staff, and managing adverse events are important considerations in developing a culture of safety for clinical trials. Strong investigatory tools, methodologies, and reporting practices help to develop the necessary infrastructure for a safe research environment for clinical trial participants. Knowing to whom to report adverse events and knowing when to report are also important factors in developing a culture of safety in human research.

References

Department of Health and Human Services, Office for Protection from Research Risks. *Institutional Review Board Guidebook*. (Chap. III, Sec. E., "Monitoring and Observation.") Washington, D.C.: U.S. Government Printing Office, 1993.

Department of Health and Human Services, Office of Inspector General. *Institutional Review Boards: A Time for Reform*. OEI-01-97-00193. Rockville, Md.: Department of Health and Human Services, June 1998.

Department of Health and Human Services, Office of Inspector General. *Protecting Human Research Subjects: Status of Recommendations*. OEI-01-97-00197. [http://oig.hhs.gov/oei/reports/oei-01-97-00197.pdf]. Apr. 2000.

Department of Health and Human Services, Office for Human Research Protections. *Guidance on Continuing Review*. [http://www.hhs.gov/ohrp/humansubjects/guidance/contrev2002.htm]. July 11, 2002.

Food and Drug Administration. *Guidance for Clinical Trial Sponsors on the Establishment and Operation of Clinical Trial Data Monitoring Committees*. Draft Guidance. Rockville, Md.: Food and Drug Administration, Nov. 2001.

National Institutes of Health. *Policy for Data and Safety Monitoring*. [http://www.nih.gov/grants/guide/notice-files/not98-084.html]. June 10, 1998.

National Institutes of Health. *Guidance on Reporting Adverse Events to Institutional Review Boards for NIH-Supported Multicenter Clinical Trials*. [http://grants.nih.gov/grants/guide/notice-files/not99-107.html]. June 11, 1999.

National Institutes of Health. *Further Guidance on Data and Safety Monitoring for Phase I and Phase II Trials*. OD-00-038. [http://grants1.nih.gov/grants/guide/notice-files/not98-084.html]. June 5, 2000.

CHAPTER ELEVEN

MEDICAL ERROR REPORTING

Maintaining Confidentiality in the Face of Litigation

Frederick Robinson
Lara E. Parkin

According to a recent survey by the University of Colorado Health Sciences Center, just 32 percent of physicians nationwide support the creation of a national agency to address the problem of medical errors (Robinson and others, 2002). Nearly all physicians agree, however, that fear of malpractice lawsuits is a barrier to error reporting, and about 90 percent say that greater legal safeguards are necessary for a mandatory reporting system to be successful. At the same time, a recent study has revealed that adverse drug events represented 6.3 percent of one medical insurer's malpractice claims and that 73 percent of these events were deemed preventable (Rothschild and others, 2002).

In the case of medical error reporting, there are grounds for concern that sharing data on medical errors with the government or an accrediting agency will waive any privilege that may have protected that information from discovery. Under Rule 26(b)(1) of the Federal Rules of Civil Procedure, and similar state rules, parties may obtain discovery regarding any matter "not privileged." Privileges recognized in discovery include the marital communications privilege, the attorney-client privilege, the attorney–work product privilege, and in most states, the physician-patient privilege. Generally, privileges are waived when the holder of the privilege shares privileged information with a third party (see, for example, *United States* v. *AT&T,* 1980). This chapter will explore the ways in which evidentiary privileges may attach to medical error reports and related records, including peer review documents, and will examine other mechanisms through which medical records can be kept confidential in the face of litigation.

Evidentiary Protections at the State Level

State-specific rules regarding what can and cannot be used as evidence in litigation are found in state laws regarding medical error and adverse-event reporting, state freedom of information acts, and state laws defining physician-patient privilege and giving protection to peer review information.

Medical Error and Adverse-Event Reporting

A number of states now require the reporting of medical errors and adverse events and offer this information some protection from discovery.

Requirements for Reporting Medical Errors and Adverse Events. According to the National Academy for State Health Policy (Rosenthal, Riley, and Booth, 2000), fifteen states require health care providers to report medical errors: Colorado, Florida, Kansas, Massachusetts, Nebraska, New Jersey, New York, Ohio, Pennsylvania, Rhode Island, South Carolina, South Dakota, Tennessee, Texas, and Washington. In August of 2002, Nevada joined these states when its governor signed a medical error reporting requirement into law as part of a medical liability reform package. Some of the remaining states, however, have not codified their requirements. And some states and the District of Columbia encourage but do not require health care providers to report medical errors and adverse events. These states include Georgia, New Mexico, North Carolina, Oregon, and Wyoming. Health care providers in this latter group of states can avoid disclosure of medical error data simply by refusing to participate in the voluntary state data collection efforts.

Protection from Discovery. Of the states that have codified their reporting requirements, several also protect medical error report information from discovery, through language that is part of the reporting requirement statute or regulation. For example, the reports and records collected under the Kansas statute are not subject to discovery, subpoena, or "other means of legal compulsion" and are not admissible in any civil legal action other than a disciplinary proceeding by the appropriate state licensing agency (*Kan. Stat. Ann.* § 65-4925, 2004). Similarly, Florida protects adverse incident reports from discovery or admission in "any civil or administrative action, except in disciplinary proceedings by the agency or appropriate regulatory board" (*Fla. Stat.* § 395.0197[13], 2004). Interestingly, these statutes do not appear to prohibit the use of medical error and adverse event reports in criminal proceedings.

A somewhat more restrictive approach has been taken by the state of Washington, which not only protects the reports but also does not allow any person who was present at a committee meeting where medical error reports were discussed to testify in any civil action regarding the content of the reports or the proceedings of the committee. An individual, however, may testify to any matter about which he has independent firsthand knowledge. Again, privileges in criminal proceedings are not discussed in the Washington rule (*Wash. Rev. Code* § 70.41.200[3], 2004). Similarly restrictive is the Colorado statute, which presumably does not apply only to civil actions because it is worded broadly to include all legal actions. This statute protects medical error reports from "subpoena, search warrant, discovery proceedings, or otherwise." Colorado law does, however, make investigation summaries available to the public. These summaries list complaints against health care facilities and the conclusions reached by the health department. The summaries do not identify the patient or the health care professional named in the full report (*Colo. Rev. Stat.* § 25-1-124[4]-[6], 2004).

Other states do not provide such comprehensive protection. For example, Pennsylvania generally protects medical error reports from disclosure "unless otherwise ordered by a court for good cause shown" (28 *Pa. Code* § 51.3[i], 2004). The rest of the states that mandate reporting of medical errors do not specifically protect medical error data from discovery. Nonetheless, this information may be protected under a state freedom of information act or by physician-patient privilege, as discussed later in this chapter.

Example of State Medical Error Reporting Laws.

- *Colorado (Colo. Rev. Stat.* § 25-1-124, 2004). Colorado health care facilities must report to the Department of Public Health and Environment any occurrence that results in the death of a patient from an unexplained cause or other suspicious circumstance. Licensed health care facilities also must report certain serious injuries; patients who are missing for more than eight hours; physical, sexual, or verbal abuse of a patient; patient neglect; misappropriation of patient property; diversion of patient drugs; and the malfunction or intentional or accidental misuse of patient care equipment. Colorado's purpose behind collecting this information is to make it available to the public to aid individuals in the "difficult task of choosing a health care facility." To that end, after redacting patient identifying information, Colorado will publicly release investigation summaries, complaints against particular facilities, and a listing of deficiency citations issued against each health care facility.

- *Florida (Fla. Stat. § 395.0197, 2004).* Licensed health care facilities in Florida are required to notify the state Agency for Health Care Administration of adverse events. Adverse events include death, brain or spinal injury, the performance of a surgical procedure on the wrong patient, the performance of the wrong surgical procedure on a patient, and the performance of a wrong-site surgical procedure on a patient. Facilities must report serious patient injuries of a volatile nature within twenty-four hours, individual serious adverse incidents within fifteen days, and all incidents identified throughout the year in an annual report. Florida will use this information to ensure proper care at its licensed facilities and may initiate disciplinary action against a facility or health care provider based on these reports. Furthermore, Florida will publish an annual report summarizing adverse incidents, malpractice claims, and disciplinary actions. The law provides no specific privilege.
- *Kansas (Kan. Stat. Ann. § 65-4921 et seq., 2004).* In Kansas, reportable incidents include any act by a health care provider that is below the applicable standard of care and that has a reasonable probability of causing injury to the patient or that may be grounds for disciplinary action by the appropriate licensing agency. If the reportable incident occurs in a medical care facility, the report shall be made to the facility's risk manager, who will refer the report to the appropriate peer review committee. The peer review committee will investigate and take appropriate action. The committee must report to the appropriate state licensing agency any finding that the health care provider acted below the applicable standard of care.
- *Massachusetts (105 Code of Mass. Regs. § 130.331, 2004).* Hospitals must report serious incidents and accidents to the Department of Public Health immediately, by telephone. Serious incidents and accidents include fire, suicide, serious criminal acts, strikes by hospital employees, and serious physical injury to patients resulting from accidents or unknown causes. Hospitals must file written reports on other serious incidents with the department within one week of the occurrence of the incident. The regulations do not specify what the department will do with the reports or whether these reports are protected from discovery.
- *New York (N.Y. Pub. Health Law, § 2805-l, 2004).* After conducting an investigation, which should take no more than thirty days, the hospital has twenty-four hours to provide the Department of Health with a copy of an incident report. Incidents subject to investigation and reporting include patient deaths and impairments due to causes other than those related to the natural course of illness, fires, medical equipment malfunction, and poisoning. Other incidents, including strikes, natural disasters, and emergencies, need to be reported but not investigated.

- *Pennsylvania (28 Pa. Code.* § 51.3, 2004). Health care facilities must report to the Department of Health events that seriously compromise quality and patient safety. Such events include deaths due to injuries, suicide, or unusual circumstances; deaths due to malnutrition, dehydration, or sepsis; deaths or serious injuries due to a medication error; surgery performed on the wrong patient or body part; and complaints of patient abuse. The Department of Health will use the information only to enforce its responsibilities and will not publish or release the information except pursuant to a court order.
- *South Carolina* (61-16 *S.C. Code of Regs.* § 206.2, 2004). In order to meet licensing requirements, South Carolina hospitals and institutional general infirmaries must keep accident and incident reports. Incident reports include medication errors and adverse drug reactions. Hospitals must report incidents that result in death or serious injury to the Department of Health Licensing within ten days of their occurrence.
- *Tennessee (Tenn. Rules* § 1200-8-1-.11, 2004). Hospitals must report incidents of an unusual nature to the Tennessee Department of Human Services. Such incidents include a fire in a hospital, the burning of a patient, suspected patient abuse, or an accident that causes injury to a patient. The incident will be investigated first within the hospital, which will then forward the incident report to the department within five working days of the incident.
- *Washington (Wash. Rev. Code* § 70.41.200, 2004). Every hospital must maintain a quality improvement program that includes the maintenance and collection of information concerning "negative health care outcomes and incidents injurious to patients." The state Health Department, in conjunction with its licensing responsibilities, will review and audit the records of the quality improvement committee. These records are specifically protected from discovery by the statute.

JCAHO Reporting Requirements: Often Complementing or Replacing State Requirements

As of February 2001, forty-six states had incorporated Joint Commission on Accreditation of Healthcare Organizations (JCAHO) accreditation standards into their hospital licensing requirements. The only states that had not done so were Hawaii, Kentucky, New Jersey, and Oklahoma. Some states look to JCAHO accreditation of other facilities as well for appropriate standards. These facilities include ambulatory care centers (eighteen states), behavioral health centers (forty-five states), home care agencies (twenty states), laboratories (twenty-eight states), long-term care facilities (fourteen states), and health care networks (twenty-one states).

The states that have incorporated JCAHO accreditation standards, have done so to varying degrees. For example, under the *Texas Health & Safety Code* (§ 222.024), a hospital licensed by the Texas Department of Health is not subject to annual licensing inspections as long as the hospital maintains JCAHO accreditation. In contrast, Pennsylvania gives credit for JCAHO inspections but does not rely exclusively on them. Pennsylvania requires its hospitals to be surveyed and licensed every two years, whereas JCAHO conducts voluntary accreditation surveys only every three years. Furthermore, JCAHO surveys do not cover certain standards specific to Pennsylvania regulations. Therefore, for those hospitals that participate in JCAHO surveys, the Pennsylvania Department of Health conducts residual surveys, taking into account JCAHO results and surveying the remaining requirements.

To maintain JCAHO accreditation, medical facilities must comply with the JCAHO sentinel event policy. This policy, implemented in 1996, is designed to help health care organizations identify sentinel events and take action to prevent their recurrence. A sentinel event, reviewable by JCAHO, is "an unexpected occurrence involving death or serious physical or psychological injury, or the risk thereof." Such events are called *sentinel* because they signal the need for immediate investigation and response. JCAHO encourages but does not require health care organizations to report sentinel events to JCAHO. In the absence of voluntary reporting, JCAHO may become aware of a sentinel event by some other means, such as communication from a patient, family member, or employee of the organization or through the media. In any case, if JCAHO becomes aware of a reviewable sentinel event, JCAHO expects the organization to prepare and submit a "thorough and credible" root cause analysis. A root cause analysis focuses primarily on systems and processes, not individual performance. The root cause analysis leads to an action plan, under which the organization implements steps to reduce future risks and monitors the effectiveness of those improvements. The organization must complete the necessary documents within forty-five days of a sentinel event of which JCAHO is aware. JCAHO then will review the analysis and action plan to determine whether they are acceptable. If the submission is not acceptable, the organization is at risk of being placed on *accreditation watch* by the JCAHO Accreditation Committee and ultimately could lose its accreditation.

JCAHO is not a governmental entity but a private accrediting body. Thus the protection that may be offered to medical records by state freedom of information acts (discussed later in this chapter) does not apply to information that medical organizations share with JCAHO. Arguably, sharing this information with JCAHO destroys any applicable state law privilege. Most states have not addressed the protection of medical information shared with JCAHO from legal discovery. Louisiana, however, has specifically addressed this data protection issue. A

Louisiana statute protects medical information including records, notes, data, studies, and proceedings of hospital committees, peer review committees, and nationally recognized improvement agencies or commissions (*La. Rev. Stat.* § 13:3715.3, 2004). The Louisiana statute goes so far as to mention JCAHO as an organization whose records are exempt from discovery or court subpoenas. Because, however, statutory protection for JCAHO records is the exception rather than the rule, JCAHO itself has taken precautions to keep information confidential.

JCAHO believes that concerns about the disclosure of personal health care information seriously threaten the quality of health care. Therefore JCAHO keeps information received or developed during the accreditation process confidential. This includes compliance information, sentinel event reports, root cause analyses, and accreditation committee minutes and agenda materials. Under normal procedures, handling of any submitted root cause analysis and action plan is restricted to specially trained staff in accordance with procedures designed to protect the confidentiality of the documents. In fact the original root cause analysis is always returned to the medical facility and any copies are shredded. Also, once the action plan has been implemented to JCAHO's satisfaction, the action plan is returned to the organization.

To further confidentiality and promote compliance, JCAHO gives medical facilities a choice of method for sentinel event reporting. Each method offers an increasing degree of confidentiality protection for organizations that are uncomfortable with the prospect of giving JCAHO sensitive and potentially discoverable information. Alternative 1 permits the organization to schedule an appointment for an organizational representative to bring the root cause analysis and other sentinel event–related documents to JCAHO headquarters for review and to take all these documents away when he or she leaves. In this way organizational representatives have a level of comfort that their documents have not been circulated or copied to unknown persons. Alternative 2 permits the organization to request an on-site review of the root cause analysis and other sentinel event–related documents. Upon receiving such a request, JCAHO will schedule a surveyor to visit the organization for the purpose of reviewing the root cause analysis and related documents. No copies of these documents will be retained by JCAHO. Alternative 3 permits the organization to request an on-site visit by a JCAHO surveyor who will conduct interviews and review relevant documentation about the findings of the root cause analysis without actually reviewing the root cause analysis. The surveyor will, however, review the action plan resulting from the root cause analysis and conduct on-site interviews. As in Alternative 2, no copy of the root cause analysis or action plan will be retained by JCAHO. Finally, Alternative 4 provides the ultimate in confidentiality. The chief executive officer of the organization electing Alternative 4 is asked to sign an affirmation statement indicating that he or she has, on behalf of the organization:

1. Considered the relevant statutes, existing protective privileges, and case law in reaching the conclusion to proceed with Alternative 4
2. Considered the other alternatives for sharing sentinel event–related information with JCAHO, and has concluded that the use of any of these other alternatives may waive existing confidentiality protections for this information
3. Determined that the organization has completed a thorough and credible root cause analysis for the event under review

Upon receiving a request under Alternative 4, JCAHO will schedule a surveyor to visit the organization. The on-site review process will involve interviews with the organization leaders and staff, a review of otherwise discoverable factual information about the sentinel event (including medical records), and a review of other relevant documentation. The surveyor will not review the root cause analysis or the resulting action plan. JCAHO may request additional information from the organization if its accreditation committee finds that the results of the on-site review are inconclusive in determining the acceptability of the organization's response to the sentinel event.

Freedom of Information Acts and Access to Medical Error Reports

State freedom of information acts may affect the confidentiality and privilege of medical error reports; however, some states exempt medical records from disclosure under freedom of information acts.

How Freedom of Information Acts May Compromise Confidentiality and Privilege. Generally, freedom of information or open records acts allow citizens to request any public information that a governmental entity keeps. For example, in Vermont any "person may inspect or copy any public record or document of a public agency, on any day other than a Saturday, Sunday or a legal holiday" (1 *Vt. Stat. Ann.* § 316, 2001). In Alabama every "citizen has a right to inspect and take a copy of any public writing of [the] state" (*Ala. Code* § 36-12-40, 2001). In Hawaii, "government records are open to public inspection unless access is restricted or closed by law" (*Haw. Rev. Stat.* § 92F-11, 2000). Arguably, "government records" could include information gathered by the state under a medical error reporting system. Therefore a citizen conceivably could walk into the state Health Department and request the medical error reports from a particular hospital or concerning a particular group of patients.

Protections from Disclosure Under Freedom of Information Acts. Fortunately, however, this scenario is not generally possible. Although the grant of access to public documents is typically broad, most of these statutes include long lists of exclusions from the general rule. Commonly excluded from public access are medical records.

States exempt medical records from disclosure under freedom of information acts in different ways. Approximately half the states specifically exempt medical records from disclosure. Some states do this by defining a public record in such a way as to exclude medical records. Others exempt medical records through a separate exemption provision. However, most of these statutes still permit disclosure in the face of a court order. Other states protect medical records by instructing the record custodian to engage in a balancing test, weighing the privacy expectations of the individuals named in the records with the public's right to know. The record custodian does not consider the institution's expectation of privacy in the records. A minority of states discuss exemption in terms of other evidentiary privileges. In other words, if the information in the records is protected by the physician-patient or peer review privilege of that state, the record itself is protected from disclosure. A few states do not discuss the protection of personal information in their freedom of information acts. In these states an analysis of whether sharing the information in the medical records violates the privilege between a physician and a patient is necessary.

Table 11.1 lists the states that have a freedom of information act, or an equivalent law, and the type of protection from disclosure offered to medical records under the statute. Although medical records may find protection under a state's physician-patient privilege (discussed later in this chapter), the scope of this table is solely the protection offered under each state's freedom of information act. States with mandatory reporting requirements are listed in bold type.

Physician-Patient Privilege

In the common law, no privilege between physicians and patients is recognized, and this is the rule in the absence of a statute. In 1828, New York became the first state to enact the privilege by statute, owing to a belief that people might be discouraged from obtaining medical help if they feared their communications to a physician might be publicly disclosed (*Williams* v. *Roosevelt Hospital,* 1985). Indeed, every state has enacted a law making certain communications between health professionals and patients privileged. This privilege, being statutory, can be modified or withdrawn. Although all states have some form of privilege, some of these laws are applicable only to psychiatrists or psychotherapists. The states that grant this privilege only to psychotherapist-patient communications are Alabama (*Ala. Rules of*

TABLE 11.1. STATES WITH A FREEDOM OF INFORMATION (OR EQUIVALENT) ACT.

State	Specific Protection of Medical Records by Exemption Clause?	Medical Records Excluded from the Definition of a Public Record?	Protection Granted Through Balancing of Privacy and Disclosure Interests?
Alabama	N	N	Maybe—judicial precedent
Alaska	Y	N	N/A
Arizona	N	N	Maybe—judicial precedent
Arkansas	Y	N	N/A
California	Y—if an invasion of personal privacy	N	N/A
Colorado	**Y**	**N**	**N/A**
Connecticut	Y—if an invasion of personal privacy	N	N/A
Delaware	N	Y—if disclosure constitutes an invasion of personal privacy	N/A
District of Columbia	Y—if clearly an unwarranted invasion of personal privacy	N	N/A
Florida	**Y—if the medical record of an agency employee or if furnished subject to housing assistance program**	**N**	**N/A**
Georgia	Y—if an invasion of personal privacy	N	N/A
Hawaii	N	N	If disclosure is an unwarranted invasion of personal privacy
Idaho	N	N	N
Illinois	Y—if a government agency provided services	N	N/A
Indiana	Y	N	N/A
Iowa	Y	N	N/A
Kansas	**Y**	**N**	**N/A**

TABLE 11.1. (*CONTINUED*)

State	Specific Protection of Medical Records by Exemption Clause?	Medical Records Excluded from the Definition of a Public Record?	Protection Granted Through Balancing of Privacy and Disclosure Interests?
Kentucky	N	N	If disclosure is a clearly unwarranted invasion of personal privacy
Louisiana	N	N	N
Maine	N	N	N
Maryland	Y	N	N/A
Massachusetts	N	Y	N/A
Michigan	Y	N	N/A
Minnesota	N	N	N
Missouri	N	N	N
Montana	N	N	Where the individual privacy interest clearly exceeds the merits of public disclosure
Nebraska	**N**	**N**	**N**
Nevada	**N**	**N**	**N**
New Hampshire	Y	N	N/A
New Jersey	**N**	**N**	**N**
New Mexico	Y—if the individual is confined to an institution	N	N/A
New York	**Y**	**N**	**N/A**
North Carolina	N	N	N
North Dakota	Y—if the record concerns a public employee or state university student at a university clinic	N	N
Ohio	**N**	**Y**	**N/A**
Oklahoma	N	N	N

(Continued)

TABLE 11.1.   STATES WITH A FREEDOM OF INFORMATION (OR EQUIVALENT) ACT. (*CONTINUED*)

State	Specific Protection of Medical Records by Exemption Clause?	Medical Records Excluded from the Definition of a Public Record?	Protection Granted Through Balancing of Privacy and Disclosure Interests?
Oregon	N	N	If public disclosure constitutes an unreasonable invasion of privacy
Pennsylvania	N	N	N
Rhode Island	N	Y	N/A
South Carolina	N	Y	N/A
South Dakota	N	N	N
Tennessee	Y	N	N/A
Texas	Only if the record is considered confidential by law	N	N
Vermont	N	N	N
Virginia	Y	N	N/A
Washington	Y	N	N/A
West Virginia	Y—if an unreasonable invasion of privacy	N	N/A
Wisconsin	N	N	N

Evid. 503, 1995), Connecticut (*Conn. Gen. Stat. Ann.* § 52-146, 1989), Florida (*Fla. Stat.* § 90.503, 1992), Georgia (*Ga. Code Ann.* § 24-9-21, 1995), Kentucky (*Ky. Rules of Evid.* 507, 1992), Maryland (9 *Md. Code Ann.* § 109, 2000), Massachusetts (*Mass. Gen. Laws* § 233:20B, 1995), South Carolina (*S.C. Code Ann.* § 19-11-95, 1995), Tennessee (*Tenn. Code* § 24-1-207, 2000), and West Virginia (*W. Va. Code* § 27-3-1, 2001). Most states limit these privileges to civil proceedings. No state allows the patient to claim the privilege where the patient's physical or mental condition is an element of the claim or defense. Most states' definition of *physician* is broad enough to include licensed psychiatrists but not counselors. A *physician* is commonly defined as one who is licensed to "practice medicine" (see, for example, *Kan. Stat.* § 60-427[2], 1992).

In most cases where a physician-patient privilege exists, that privilege has been held to apply to hospital records (*American Jurisprudence*, 2004). For example, in *Payne*

v. *Howard* (1977) the District of Columbia District Court held that a dentist need not comply with a request for discovery of third-party patient medical records. In *Payne*, the plaintiff sued his dentist for malpractice. In an effort to prove his case, the plaintiff requested the medical records of other patients for whom the dentist had provided the same treatment. The issue was whether those medical records were discoverable. The *Payne* court held they were not. The court held that because communications between a doctor and his patient were privileged under District of Columbia law, the medical records, which "necessarily reflect communications made by patients to defendant . . . in confidence," fell "squarely within the bounds of the statutory protection." Therefore the plaintiff was not allowed to review the third-party patient records.

In other cases, however, courts have held that with the proper precautions, third-party medical information is discoverable. In *Cochran* v. *St. Paul Fire and Marine Ins. Co.* (1995), the district court found that medication incident reports, kept by a hospital, were discoverable where the names of the nonparty patients were deleted from the reports. In this malpractice action for injuries sustained after an intravenous delivery of medication, the plaintiff requested redacted copies of "medication incident reports." The defendant claimed that the reports were protected under the privilege set forth in Arkansas Rule of Evidence 503, dealing with patient privileges. The court disagreed, finding that the medication incident reports were discoverable in redacted form. Specifically, the *Cochran* court reasoned that the "defendant's concern regarding the patient privilege is removed by the phrasing of plaintiff's document request. Plaintiff requests only redacted copies which omit the patient's name." As a result the plaintiff was able to review the medication incident reports. Using similar reasoning the Florida Supreme Court held in *Amente* v. *Newman* (1995) that the patient's right to privacy in his or her medical records was satisfied by the trial judge's requirement that all identifying information be redacted from the medical records. In *Amente*, the plaintiff sued her doctor for malpractice because her child was injured during delivery. Because the plaintiff was morbidly obese, her contention was that the delivery required special precautions. Therefore she sought the medical records of other obese obstetric patients to see whether the physician used a different delivery method with those patients. The issue was whether the release of those medical records invaded the third-party patients' constitutional right to privacy. The court held that it did not. In *Amente*, the plaintiff specifically requested that all patient identifying information be redacted from the medical records before production. That precaution was enough in the court's opinion to protect the privacy of the other patients, who were not parties to the suit. Thus the plaintiff was able to review the medical records after the patient identifying information was redacted. In his concurrence, Justice Overton cautioned that although redaction of patient names may have been enough to protect privacy in this instance, in other circumstances, "such as where the doctor serves a more sparsely populated area, more information may have to be redacted from the records to ensure absolute anonymity."

Although most jurisdictions apply the physician-patient privilege to medical records, some do not. Several jurisdictions extend protection only to testimony that reveals confidential medical information. For example, the Iowa Supreme Court found that the "mental health professional–patient privilege" did not bar disclosure of patient records because the privilege in Iowa is "limited to disclosure of confidential communication by the giving of testimony" (*McMaster* v. *Board of Psychology Examiners*, 1993). Although the *McMaster* court found the state privilege statute inapplicable, it also found that the constitutional right to privacy should extend to medical records and protected the records from disclosure on that basis.

In fact a constitutional right to privacy often factors into state court analyses. In *Berger* v. *Lutheran General Hospital* (2001), the plaintiff alleged that the hospital's negligence in treating her leg injury ultimately resulted in an amputation that would not otherwise have been necessary. In the course of litigation the plaintiff filed an emergency motion to bar *ex parte* communication between the hospital's counsel and those members of its medical staff, agents, and employees who provided health care to plaintiff but were not named as defendants. One of the plaintiff's arguments was that such intercompany disclosures violated her right to privacy under the Illinois constitution because "there is nothing [plaintiff], or any patient, could do to keep her doctors and nurses from talking to hospital counsel or risk management about any care they ever provided to her." The court, however, found no violation of the plaintiff's right to privacy. In its analysis the court reasoned that only unreasonable invasions of privacy are barred by the Illinois constitution. The court found it significant that in the modern hospital setting, health care services are provided by a wide array of hospital personnel. Therefore the court concluded that "a hospital patient could not reasonably expect a member of the hospital's medical staff, or the hospital's agents and employees, to refrain from discussing [within the limited community of the hospital organization] the medical care provided to the patient." Because the hospital's internal disclosure of medical records was not, in the court's view, an unreasonable invasion of privacy, the court denied plaintiff's emergency motion.

It is important to remember that as illustrated in *Cochran* and *Amente*, regardless of whether the physician-patient privilege applies to medical records, the medical care providers in question had no privacy interest in the medical records. The privilege in these cases belonged to the patients alone, and only patient information was required to be redacted from the records. Generally, physicians can claim the privilege but only on behalf of the patient. In fact the *Cochran* court refused the defendant's request that the names of the health professionals involved in the cases be redacted from the medication incident reports. Some states specifically address this concept in their privilege statutes. For example, the Nevada statute states, "The person who was the doctor may claim the privilege but only on behalf of the patient" (*Nev. Rev. Stat.* § 49.235[2], 2004). New Mexico (*N.M. R. Evid.* § 11-504[C], 2004), South Dakota (*S.D. Code* § 19-13-8, 2004), and Texas (*Tex. Rules of Evid.* 509[d][2], 2004), among others, use similar wording in their privilege statutes. Therefore a hospital's release of medical error data to governmental or accrediting agencies cannot, in theory, waive an evidentiary privilege held by a patient. It is likely, however, that patients at many institutions unknowingly sign away their privilege by authorizing, upon their admittance to the medical institution, the sharing of medical records under these circumstances. In Mississippi such a waiver is implied by statute (*Miss. Code* § 13-1-21[2], 2004).

Indeed, a close reading of one's particular state privilege statute is required, because some state courts have held that statutory privileges, such as the physician-patient privilege, can be waived only in the manner specified by the statute. For example, in *Nielson* v. *Bryson* (1970), the plaintiff contended that under the Oregon statute, "consent to examine medical records is not deemed to have been given by the mere filing of an action for personal injuries, but only if and when a patient, as a party to the action, 'offers himself as a witness.'" The Supreme Court of Oregon agreed. Specifically, the court found that an "accelerated waiver" of the physician-patient privilege, where courts refuse to docket personal injury cases until the plaintiff has agreed to waive the privilege for pretrial discovery, goes against the legislative intent of the Oregon statute.

Table 11.2 summarizes the status of physician-patient privilege in the states as of November 30, 2001.

Protection of Peer Review Information

Many states require that individual hospitals provide peer review of the professional practices within the hospital for the purpose of improving the quality of care and reducing medical errors. States developed peer review statutes in response to the enactment of the federal Health Care Quality Improvement Act of 1986 (HCQIA), in which Congress sought to curtail the occurrence of medical malpractice by inhibiting the state-to-state movement of physicians who failed to disclose their prior damaging or incompetent acts. Nearly all of the fifty states have enacted peer review statutes in keeping with the HCQIA, but subtle differences

TABLE 11.2. PHYSICIAN-PATIENT PRIVILEGE BY STATE, NOVEMBER 30, 2001.

State	Physician Privilege?	Psychotherapist Privilege?	Privilege Specifically Limited to Civil Proceedings?	Physician or Psychotherapist Specifically Allowed to Invoke on Behalf of Patient?
Alabama	N	Y	Does not apply for criminal insanity defense	Y
Alaska	Y	Y	Only psychotherapist privilege applies in criminal proceeding	Y
Arizona	Y	N	Y	N
Arkansas	Y	Y	N	Y
California	Y	N	Y	Y
Colorado	Y	Y	N	N
Connecticut	N	Y	N	N
Delaware	Y	Y	N—but not applicable to child abuse proceedings	Y
District of Columbia	Y	Y	N—but not applicable to murder cases	N
Florida	N	Y	N	Y
Georgia	N	Y	N	N
Hawaii	Y	N	N	Y
Idaho	Y	N	Y	N
Illinois	Y	Y	N—but not applicable to murder cases	N
Indiana	Y	N	N	N
Iowa	Y	Y	N	N
Kansas	Y	N	Limited to civil actions and misdemeanors	N
Kentucky	N	Y	N	N
Louisiana	Y	Y	N	Y
Maine	Y	Y	N	Y
Maryland	N	Y	N	N
Massachusetts	N	Y	N	N
Michigan	Y	N	N	N
Minnesota	Y	Y	N	N

TABLE 11.2. (CONTINUED)

State	Physician Privilege?	Psychotherapist Privilege?	Privilege Specifically Limited to Civil Proceedings?	Physician or Psychotherapist Specifically Allowed to Invoke on Behalf of Patient?
Mississippi	Y	N	N	N
Missouri	Y	Y	N	N
Montana	Y	Y	N	N
Nebraska	Y	Y	N	Y
Nevada	Y	Y	N	Y
New Hampshire	Y	N	N	N
New Jersey	Y	Y	N	N
New Mexico	Y	Y	N	Y
New York	Y	Y	N	N
North Carolina	Y	Y	N	N
North Dakota	Y	Y	N	Y
Ohio	Y	N	N	N
Oklahoma	Y	Y	N	Y
Oregon	Y	Y	Y	Y
Pennsylvania	Y	Y	N	N
Rhode Island	Y	N	N	N
South Carolina	N	Y	N	N
South Dakota	Y	Y	N	Y
Tennessee	N	Y	N	N
Texas	Y	Y	Y	Y
Utah	Y	N	Y	N
Vermont	Y	Y	N	N
Virginia	Y	Y	N	N
Washington	Y	N	Y	N
West Virginia	N	Y	N	N
Wisconsin	Y	Y	N—but not applicable to murder or child abuse cases	Y
Wyoming	Y	N	N	N

exist in the information that each state deems confidential, and the statutes are usually strictly construed.

Peer Review Privilege of Committees. State statutes usually assign the peer review confidentiality privilege to committees. Routinely protected committees include medical staff committees, such as committees that review morbidity and mortality, executive committees that review performance, and multidisciplinary committees that evaluate a hospital's quality of care (see, for example, *Wall* v. *Ohio Permanente Medical Group,* 1997; *Mulder* v. *VanKersen,* 1994; *Santa Rosa Memorial Hospital* v. *Superior Court,* 1985). Some states grant confidentiality to peer review committees composed of the entire medical staff (*Corrigan* v. *Methodist Hospital,* 1995). Other states require that the committee for which the privilege is sought operate pursuant to bylaws approved by the hospital board (*Suwannee County Hospital Corp.* v. *Meeks,* 1985). In *University of Texas Health Science Center* v. *Jordan* (1985), the work of a quality of care review committee established by a medical school pursuant to its bylaws was found to be privileged.

The immunity enjoyed by committee members as a group does not necessarily extend to an individual committee member acting independently, and committees that do not evaluate patient care are not entitled to the peer review privilege. Further, any portion of committee work that does not pertain to patient care can be isolated and made discoverable. In fact, in *State ex rel. St. John's Mercy Medical Center* v. *Hoester* (1986), the court held that "records of meetings, conferences, or consultations may not be shielded from discovery in medical malpractice actions merely by labeling them as meetings of peer review committees." Missouri's peer review statute establishes privilege for the work of groups of health care professionals that focuses on the quality and utilization of health care. Meetings for any other purpose or of other groups may be relevant but are not protected from discovery. The records of licensure board committees also often fall outside state peer review privilege. In some cases the committee does not satisfy the definition of a medical review committee, as in *Kutner* v. *Davenport* (1987). In other cases the records are discoverable due to a party's interest in obtaining the records, which were public records at common law (*Beck* v. *Bluestein,* 1984).

Peer Review Privilege of Documents. Typically, statutory privilege is assigned to documents that are produced primarily or solely for use during the peer review process. Documents that are available and sought from original sources, however, remain discoverable. Many state statutes recognize as an original source the testimony of a peer review committee member who possesses personal knowledge not obtained in the peer review process, but courts often will bar testimony by a witness whose knowledge could derive from both personal and peer review experience (*Fox* v. *Kramer,* 1999).

Committee minutes, records, and guidelines are generally privileged. For example, in *Kappas* v. *Chestnut Lodge* (1983), transcripts of hospital staff conferences held to discuss a particular patient were excluded from evidence as files of a "medical review committee," under Maryland's peer review statute (*Md. Code Ann., Health Occ.* § 14-601, 1981). Likewise, in *Ekstrom* v. *Temple* (1990) the hospital's infection control guidelines were held to be privileged under the Illinois Medical Studies Act.

The assignment of privilege to documents created by committees that serve purposes in addition to peer review varies from state to state. For example, in *Santa Rosa Memorial Hospital* v. *Superior Court* (1985) the court held that a hospital's infection control committee was a medical staff committee and that its records qualified for protection from discovery, even though a majority of its members were not physicians. Somewhat differently, in *Sakosko* v. *Memorial Hospital* (1988), the court considered pathology reports and an infection control physician's consultation report privileged even though they were prepared not for a peer review committee but for a hospital's environmental services infection control committee. The court reasoned that the committee worked on quality control and medical study that improve patient care. In contrast the court in *Babcock* v. *Bridgeport Hospital* (1999) found that documents created by a peer review infection control committee were not afforded peer review privilege because they were not created primarily for peer review committee proceedings.

Incident reports in some states also are protected by peer review privilege. In *Community Hospital of Indianapolis* v. *Medtronic* (1992) the court protected employee-generated incident reports filed with the hospital's quality assurance department for review by the director and in-house counsel. Likewise, in *Dorris* v. *Detroit Osteopathic Hospital Corp.* (1999) the privilege was extended to investigatory documents related to incident reports. In contrast, incident reports were not privileged in *Chicago Trust Co.* v. *Cook County Hospital* (1998) because the hospital failed to show that a peer review committee had requested them. Similarly, in *John C. Lincoln Hospital and Health Center* v. *Superior Court* (1989), the hospital's incident reports were filed not only in relation to quality of care but also in relation to issues not related to patient care and so were found to constitute raw data not covered by the peer review privilege.

Peer Review Statutes. In view of the differences in the state statutes and in the judicial interpretation of each statute, a careful examination of the forum state's statute and relevant case law is crucial. For each state's peer review statute, Table 11.3 lists the areas in which careful assessment of pertinent case law is particularly warranted.

TABLE 11.3.   AREAS TO ANALYZE IN STATE PEER REVIEW STATUTES.

State	Areas for Analysis
Alabama	Shareholder MDs of private corporation do not qualify as medical staff under statute.
Alaska	None found.
Arizona	Incident reports are not privileged. Peer review documents, including identity of panel members and list of documents, are privileged. Records of hospital action against defendant MDs not privileged.
Arkansas	Information about revocation of defendant MD privileges is absolutely privileged. Incident reports prepared according to policy and procedures are not privileged, even if also used in peer review.
California	Peer review committee, including infection control committees, need not be made up only of physicians to be privileged. Documents generated in subsequent investigation are not privileged. Statements made by nondefendants to peer review committee are not privileged.
Colorado	Assess hospital bylaws and operating procedures for committee's source of authority, composition, and function to determine peer review committee privilege.
Connecticut	Records of peer review proceedings, findings, and deliberations privileged if initiated at hospital request or at established committee meetings.
Delaware	Privilege extends to suits brought in another forum when the underlying transaction took place in Delaware.
District of Columbia	The key to the discoverability of materials contained in a peer review body's report is that they not owe their existence to the peer review investigation. Peer review compilations or summaries of documents that are individually available from other sources are privileged.
Florida	Date, place, and existence of peer review records are privileged. Privilege extends to depositions of defendant MDs whose knowledge was gained in peer review proceeding.
Georgia	Committee peer review function and purpose evaluated to determine privilege. Peer review records incorporated into reports to governmental agencies retain privilege.
Hawaii	Per peer review privilege; expert not required to provide documentation or testimony regarding peer review summary.
Idaho	Where peer review privilege protects board proceedings during which a defendant MD sought a second opinion, court enjoins the plaintiff from arguing noncompliance with second opinion standard of care.

TABLE 11.3. (*CONTINUED*)

State	Areas for Analysis
Illinois	No privilege for work by individual unless bylaws confer authority to act for committee. Infection control committee is privileged. Guidelines for peer review generated outside the committee are privileged. No privilege for information about the existence, date, and participants at meetings about care unless information is the substance of peer review materials. Responses to quality issues are not privileged if not generated by oversight committee.
Indiana	Modification of MD staff privileges as a result of peer review proceedings is outside the scope of peer review privilege.
Iowa	An expert who generated peer review documents can give opinion testimony that is not reliant on peer review records.
Kansas	"Disciplinary action form" is subject to balancing test of privilege versus plaintiffs' right to access. Documents from investigation subsequent to peer review are not privileged.
Kentucky	Relevant information (such as complaints) is not privileged simply because placed in peer review file; must be generated by peer review investigation to be privileged.
Louisiana	Hospital infection rate records relevant to case are not entirely privileged. Patient care evaluations by MD quality assurance committee members are privileged.
Maine	Information gathered during peer review and disclosed to a consulting MD retains privilege as part and parcel of peer review process.
Maryland	Information about staff privilege reduction due to unprofessional conduct is privileged in civil action except when the physician disputes the disciplinary action. Peer review privilege is determined by balancing hospital's need for discovery of physician's confidential peer review committee files and interest of federal antitrust laws in preserving free competition.
Massachusetts	Outside consultant's information to and conversations with peer review committee are peer review proceedings and so privileged. Incident reports that are necessary to comply with risk management and quality assurance programs are privileged. Peer review privilege turns on the purpose for which information is generated, not information content.
Michigan	Privilege turns on hospital's bylaws, rules, and regulations that define peer review committee as functioning for purpose of improvement and self-analysis.
Minnesota	Confidentiality provision can encompass all documents in peer review files, including those available from other sources. Provider data exception permits provider access to record of limitations placed on provider's staff privilege.

(Continued)

TABLE 11.3.   AREAS TO ANALYZE IN STATE PEER REVIEW STATUTES. (*CONTINUED*)

State	Areas for Analysis
Mississippi	Peer review committee records and transcripts of proceedings are privileged. Material otherwise discoverable from original sources and factual data available to the committee but not generated by or collected for the use of the committee is discoverable.
Missouri	Peer review proceedings, findings, and deliberations are privileged. Privilege applies only to groups duly appointed and designated with quality assurance purpose.
Montana	Privilege applies to records of professional training, supervision, or discipline of medical staff.
Nebraska	Peer review privilege waivable by patient and subject to court order in extraordinary circumstances. Incident reports are not privileged when prepared per standing directive.
Nevada	Occurrence reports are not necessarily covered by privilege. Only documents derived directly from peer review process are privileged.
New Hampshire	Federal Protection and Advocacy for Mentally Ill Individuals Act found not to preempt state law, which provides that records of an ambulatory care clinic's quality assurance program shall be confidential and privileged.
New Jersey	No privilege against discovery, but peer review committees are protected for actions, recommendations, or statements that they make.
New Mexico	Privilege applies to information and opinions generated exclusively for peer review. Morbidity and mortality review records are confidential as "self-critical analysis." Trial court shall compel production of confidential information that is critical to the cause of action or defense.
New York	Peer review statutes inapplicable to a malpractice action brought under the Federal Tort Claims Act. Retrospective "complication reports" are discoverable. Verbal or written statements made by a party during peer review proceeding are redacted for discovery.
North Carolina	Peer review privilege extended to committees formed pursuant to bylaws for evaluation of quality, cost, medical necessity, or credentialing, but board of trustees is not privileged. Committee must identify existing documents and their custodians.
North Dakota	No privilege for peer review records obtained from another, original source. No privilege for testimony by peer review committee member if member's knowledge was obtained outside of peer review participation.
Ohio	Privilege extends to documents of utilization review and quality assurance committees of hospital, to members and employees of such committees, and to hospital morbidity and mortality conference reports in a physician's action alleging abuse of peer review process.

TABLE 11.3. (*CONTINUED*)

State	Areas for Analysis
Oklahoma	Statements presented during peer review but based on speaker's personal knowledge are subject to disclosure.
Oregon	Hospital disciplinary committee transcripts and testimony are not admissible into evidence.
Pennsylvania	Documents used in determination of staff privileges are confidential records of peer review committee. Incident reports prepared for peer review are privileged. Incident reports prepared for patient records are not privileged because they are subject to the "original source" exception.
Rhode Island	Infection control committee records are privileged as peer review records.
South Carolina	Medical expert testimony based on information obtained independently of peer review is not privileged. MD applications for staff privileges and supporting documentation are privileged.
South Dakota	Communication by or to peer review committee about ethical or professional practice is privileged from civil or criminal, but not administrative, discovery.
Tennessee	Privilege turns not on whether committee performed a function but on whether the information was sent to peer review in furtherance of the function.
Texas	Quality and competence functions and actions of committee determine qualification of committee and its documents for privilege. Board of medical examiners privilege cannot be waived by party. Incident reports with affidavit proving peer review use are privileged; incident reports created in ordinary course of business are discoverable. Telephone logs about peer review are privileged.
Utah	Only documents prepared specifically for quality review purposes are privileged, not documents that might or could be used in the review process.
Vermont	Testimony by peer review participants about peer review process is admissible when not dependent on inadmissible peer review material.
Virginia	Medical malpractice committee is entitled to depose medical malpractice peer review member concerning deliberative process. Peer review privilege does not belong to the physician who is the subject of peer review and may not be unilaterally waived by the physician.
Washington	Guidelines, JCAHO standards, bylaws, and committee function identify privileged peer review committee, which must be regularly constituted and have duty of concurrent review and evaluation of quality of care. Information generated outside of review committee meetings otherwise available from original sources is not privileged. Incident reports filed pursuant to lawsuit are not privileged.

(Continued)

TABLE 11.3.   AREAS TO ANALYZE IN STATE PEER REVIEW
STATUTES. (*CONTINUED*)

State	Areas for Analysis
West Virginia	Material otherwise available from original sources not privileged. Hospital committee that determines staff privileges or credentials is a privileged review organization.
Wisconsin	JCAHO site surveys are equivalent to peer review and privileged. Materials about a health care provider created by peer review are privileged. Records merely presented or produced for review or evaluation are discoverable. In determining whether records are discoverable, identify persons preparing record and determine function. Hospital governing bodies are not privileged.
Wyoming	Privileged peer review can be performed by medical staff, medical society, or other outside MD organization.

Evidentiary Protections at the Federal Level

Various federal laws and regulations require medical error and adverse-event reporting and also provide some protection for such information and for medical records.

Medical Error and Adverse-Event Reporting Requirements and Protections

The CDC and the FDA manage several systems for both mandatory and voluntary adverse-event reporting.

CDC National Nosocomial Infections Surveillance System. The National Nosocomial Infections Surveillance (NNIS) system of the Centers for Disease Control and Prevention (CDC) is a voluntary reporting system, started cooperatively by the CDC and participating acute care hospitals in order to create a national database of hospital-associated infections. According to the CDC's Web site (CDC, 2003), the database is used to "describe the epidemiology of these infections, describe antimicrobial resistance trends in hospitals," and "produce hospital-associated infection rates to use for comparison purposes." The data are also used to track progress nationally in reducing infections in hospitalized, high-risk patients and are used by both participating and nonparticipating hospitals to emulate the most promising methods for detecting problems and monitoring prevention and control efforts. CDC assures participating hospitals that any information that would permit identification of any individual or institution will be held in strict confidence.

The CDC Web site explains that trained infection control personnel use standardized definitions and surveillance protocols to ensure that the data are uniformly collected. This explanation tends to show that the data will be statistically useful. However, the Web site does not explain how data will be protected. Nonetheless, under the federal Freedom of Information Act (discussed later in this chapter), it is unlikely that any data could be obtained for the purpose of legal discovery. If medical data can be obtained under the Freedom of Information Act at all, they are likely to be redacted, with identifying characteristics removed. At the beginning of 2000, approximately 315 hospitals were participating in the NNIS system.

FDA Center for Devices and Radiological Health: Manufacturer and User Facility Device Experience (MAUDE) Database.

The Food and Drug Administration (FDA), under the authority of the Safe Medical Devices Act of 1990, requires medical device user facilities, such as hospitals, ambulatory surgical facilities, nursing homes, outpatient diagnostic facilities and outpatient treatment facilities, and medical device manufacturers and importers to report certain medical device events (Public Law 101-629; 21 *C.F.R.* 803, 1990). Specifically, the FDA requires these entities to report medical device malfunctions and deaths or serious injuries caused by medical devices. The purpose behind the FDA medical device report (MDR) requirement is to protect public health by ensuring that devices are not adulterated or misbranded and that they are safe and effective for their intended use.

The FDA, in accordance with its own regulations, makes MDR data available for public disclosure (21 *C.F.R.* § 803.9). However, FDA regulations are careful to protect not only the identity of individual patients but also the identity of reporting medical device user facilities. Before disclosing any information the FDA will delete trade secret or confidential commercial information, personal medical and similar information, and the names of third parties who voluntarily submit an MDR. Similarly, except in limited situations, the FDA will not disclose the name of the device user facility that makes a report. The FDA will, however, according to the regulations, release otherwise confidential information pursuant to a final court order or as necessary in court proceedings.

Nonetheless, courts have limited discovery of MDRs in litigation. The court of appeals in *York* v. *American Medical Systems* (1998) found that the plain language of the FDA provisions does not permit automatic disclosure of personal information. According to the *York* court, even though the regulations permit disclosure during FDA proceedings or other court proceedings, the FDA is required to take precautions to ensure that it discloses no more information than is necessary under the circumstances. Furthermore, under the regulations, disclosure is permitted under a court order only when both the manufacturer and the party experiencing the adverse event are involved in the litigation. Therefore, "it follows that only parties involved in the York litigation may petition the court for a court order requiring American Medical Systems to disclose its MDRs relating to the York litigation, not MDRs relating to parties not involved in York's case." In making its decision the *York* court found that American Medical Systems had a key policy concern on its side. "The entire reporting scheme of the FDA is based on confidential reporting by manufacturers, physicians and patients. To encourage voluntary reporting, it is necessary to ensure reporters that their information will be kept in confidence and not cavalierly disclosed in various litigation." Therefore the *York* court reasoned that requiring the plaintiff to demonstrate severe hardship before MDRs are produced is reasonable. Because the plaintiff failed to demonstrate severe hardship, the court upheld the protective order.

FDA Center for Biologics Evaluation and Research: Biological Product Deviation Reporting System. The FDA Center for Biologics Evaluation and Research, Biological Product Deviation Reporting (BPDR) system requires licensed manufacturers of all biological products, unlicensed registered blood establishments, and transfusion services to report any event associated with biologics that represents a deviation in manufacturing (21 *C.F.R.* §§ 600.14, 606.171, 2004). Biologics include blood, blood components, and source plasma. A deviation in manufacturing is any event that may effect the safety, purity, or potency of a distributed product. FDA regulations require that the reports be submitted as soon as possible, but not more than forty-five days from the date the manufacturer acquires information on a reportable event. The regulations do not address the confidentiality of this information. However, as discussed later in this chapter, this information is not likely to be released under the federal Freedom of Information Act.

MedWatch. Through its MedWatch program, the FDA conducts postmarketing surveillance of medical products to identify safety concerns and take necessary action. MedWatch is a voluntary medical products reporting program. Health care professionals and consumers directly report adverse events involving medical products and product problems, including medical product errors, to this confidential and protected passive surveillance system. All reports undergo triage and are transferred to the appropriate FDA center for evaluation and entry into the appropriate FDA database. FDA centers that use this information include the Center for Drug Evaluation and Research (CDER), the Center for Biologics Evaluation and Research (CBER), the Center for Food Safety and Applied Nutrition (CFSAN), and the Center for Devices and Radiological Health (CDRH).

Ultimately, the program has four goals. First, MedWatch seeks to increase awareness of drug- and device-induced disease. Second, MedWatch looks for ways to clarify what information should and should not be reported to the FDA. Third,

MedWatch endeavors to make reporting adverse events easier by operating a single reporting system through which health care providers can alert the FDA to problems with medical products. Finally, MedWatch seeks to provide regular feedback to the health care community about medical product safety issues.

A key point to remember about MedWatch is that the FDA does not want reports of all adverse reactions and especially not the ones listed as possible side effects on a product's label. According to MedWatch director Dianne Kennedy, "All drugs have side effects. If we were to get reports of all adverse reactions, we'd be overwhelmed, making it difficult for us to focus on the issues with the most public health impact" (Henkel, 1998). Therefore the incidents reported to MedWatch should fall in one of the following categories: death, life-threatening hazard, hospitalization, disability, birth defect, miscarriage, or a condition that needs intervention to prevent permanent damage. It is not necessary, however, to prove conclusively before one makes a report that the medical product caused the adverse reaction (Henkel, 1998).

Patient Safety Task Force. The Department of Health and Human Services established the Patient Safety Task Force to coordinate and integrate data collection on medical errors and adverse events, coordinate research and analysis efforts, and promote collaboration on reducing injuries that result from medical errors. HHS hopes that the activities of the Patient Safety Task Force will contribute to HHS's efforts to reduce medical errors by 50 percent in five years. The task force is made up of representatives of four agencies: the Agency for Healthcare Research and Quality (AHRQ), the Centers for Disease Control and Prevention, the Food and Drug Administration, and the Centers for Medicare & Medicaid Services. The task force met in April 2001 to discuss such topics as collaboration between agencies, confidentiality issues, minimizing data burdens, and a proposed system for data collection. Julie Gerberding, then head of the hospital infections program at the CDC, presented the proposed federal Patient Safety Data System. The task force contracted with MEDSTAT, a health information company, to make recommendations regarding the best method for integrating information from the various agencies. In the end the task force will collect two types of data. First, AHRQ will support a series of demonstration projects to identify the causes of errors and to develop evidence-based systems for reducing errors and mitigating potential harm when they do occur. Second, data from the existing FDA and CDC reporting systems will be incorporated into the coordinated system. According to HHS, maintaining confidentiality of individual patients and providers in the reported information should be paramount.

Statutory and Regulatory Protection of Medical Records

The information in medical records is protected by a number of federal rules, regulations, and laws. Further protection may be forthcoming under a proposed Patient Safety Improvement Act.

Federal Rule of Evidence 501. According to the Federal Rules of Evidence, Rule 501, privileges are governed by courts' interpretation of the common law "in the light of reason and experience." Because nondisclosure of information to the courts is seen as a negative action, it must be justified by some balancing good. The best illustration of this is found in Wigmore's criteria (1961, § 2285, p. 527) for protecting privileged communications:

1. The communications must originate in a confidence that they will not be disclosed.
2. This element of confidentiality must be essential to the full and satisfactory maintenance of the relation between the parties.
3. The relation must be one which in the opinion of the community ought to be sedulously fostered.
4. The injury that would inure to the relation by the disclosure of the communications must be greater than the benefit thereby gained for the correct disposal of the litigation.

For example, the privilege for confidential marital communications is justified not because it is bad for courts to pry into marital secrets but because the revelation of such secrets is likely to have a destructive impact on marriages. There is no privilege for physician-patient communications under federal law, however. Arguably, this is because confidentiality is not required for a patient to show a doctor his or her symptoms when sick. Physical examination of a patient involves no communication that is endangered by a lack of confidentiality. A patient has certain symptoms whether or not that patient decides to disclose them, and the doctor is in a position to view the symptoms firsthand. However, as is discussed later, the courts have recognized a psychotherapist-patient privilege, ostensibly because that relationship does depend on open, verbal communication for effective diagnosis and treatment.

Federal Rule of Civil Procedure 26(c). On the subject of the duty to disclose during discovery, Federal Rule of Civil Procedure (FRCP) 26(c) states that "the court in the district where the deposition is to be taken may make any order which justice requires to protect a party or person from annoyance, embarrassment, oppression, or undue burden or expense, including . . . that the disclosure or discovery not be had." Before the court will issue a protective order for medical records on the basis that their disclosure would constitute embarrassment or oppression, however, FRCP 26(c) requires that the movant confer with the other affected parties in a good faith effort to resolve the discovery dispute without the need for court intervention. In fact, protective orders in litigation are often obtained by agreement between the parties. "Frequently these take the form of 'umbrella' protective orders that authorize any person producing information to designate that which is confidential as protected under the order" (Wright, Miller, and others, 1998). For example, in *Reproductive Services* v. *Walker* (1978), the U.S. Supreme Court endorsed such an agreement between the parties, fashioned to keep the identities of abortion clinic patients confidential. After approving the agreement between the parties, the *Walker* Court dissolved its stay on discovery entered in a prior proceeding. Such orders have had semiofficial endorsement since the Judicial Conference of the United States adopted the *Handbook of Procedures for the Trial of Protracted Cases* in 1960.

Privacy Act of 1974. Congress enacted the Privacy Act in order to protect the privacy of personal and financial data maintained in federal information systems (*Kimberlin* v. *Dept. of Justice,* 1986). The Privacy Act binds only federal agencies and covers only records in the possession and control of federal agencies (5 *U.S.C.* § 552a, 2000). The Privacy Act works to keep personal information from being disclosed without the individual's consent. Specifically, the Act protects medical history that contains an individual's name, identifying number or symbol, or other identifying particular assigned to the individual. The Act forbids any federal agency to disclose such information unless, among other things, a valid *need to know* exists, a *routine use* exception applies, or disclosure is made pursuant to a court order. Under the routine use exception to the Privacy Act, records that would otherwise be protected from disclosure may be discovered. Courts have defined *routine use* as the use of a record compatible with its collection purpose (*Kimberlin* v. *Dept. of Justice,* 1986). Routine uses of medical records might include the release of records to a billing contractor or to a laboratory or for other treatment or administrative uses. Legal discovery, however, is not normally compatible with the collection purpose of medical data. In fact, a Veterans Administration regulation authorizing the disclosure of information pursuant to grand jury subpoenas as "routine use" was held invalid (*Doe* v. *Stephens,* 1988).

Freedom of Information Act. The federal Freedom of Information Act (FOIA) works to allow "public access to official information unnecessarily shielded from the public view" (*Parton* v. *U.S. Department of Justice,* 1984). The idea behind the FOIA is that requiring agencies to adhere to a philosophy of full disclosure will help ensure an informed citizenry, "vital to the functioning of a democratic society" (*U.S. Department of Justice* v. *Tax Analysts*, 1988). Consistent with this purpose, the strong presumption in favor of disclosure, along with the plain language of the FOIA, places the burden on the agency to justify the withholding of any requested documents (*U.S. Department of State* v. *Ray*, 1991).

The FOIA does not, however, provide carte blanche to citizens seeking information. It also lists types of documents that are specifically exempt from disclosure, including "personnel and medical files and similar files the disclosure of which would constitute a clearly unwarranted invasion of privacy" (5 *U.S.C.* § 552[b][6], 2000). Courts have interpreted this to mean that to fall under this exemption, the files must be personnel, medical, or similar files *and* the disclosure must be an unwarranted invasion of privacy. Determining whether an invasion of privacy is unwarranted requires a balancing of private rights with public interests. An important point for the present analysis is that the courts have found no public interest in using the FOIA as a discovery tool in private litigation (see, for example, *Roberts* v. *Department of Health and Human Services*, 1988).

In *Roberts* the plaintiff requested medical questionnaires from the Department of Health and Human Services under the FOIA. HHS provided the questionnaires but redacted the names from the questionnaires. The issue for the district court was whether the plaintiff could compel HHS to release the names under FOIA. The court found that the plaintiff could not. Balancing private and public interests, the court found that there was almost no burden on the right to privacy because the questionnaires were, at best, "rudimentary" medical records. However, the court found no public interest that would be served by releasing the names because the plaintiff was "attempting to use the FOIA as a discovery tool in private litigation, a purpose for which it was never intended." Another example of a case in which the court balanced interests in applying this exemption is *U.S. Department of State* v. *Ray* (1991). In *Ray*, the Supreme Court found that immigration records could be released only after the State Department redacted personal information. In response to the plaintiff's FOIA request, the Department of State produced twenty-five documents containing information about Haitian nationals who had attempted to immigrate illegally to the United States. The State Department deleted the names from seventeen of the documents. The issue for the Court was whether these deletions were authorized by the FOIA exemption. The Court held that the redactions were proper because, as the Court had repeatedly held, "the text of the exemption requires the Court to balance the individual's right of privacy against the basic policy of opening agency action to the light of public scrutiny." When making these determinations, a court must "evaluate both the public benefit and the potential invasion of privacy by looking at the nature of the information requested and the uses to which it could be put if released to any members of the public" (*Painting Industry of Hawaii* v. *Department of the Air Force*, 1994).

Other Federal Statutes. Several other federal statutes provide protection of confidential medical information. Although these statutes do not specifically address information gathered as a function of medical error reporting, there may conceivably be overlap between information collected by a medical error reporting program and information protected by the following statutes.

The Social Security Act protects medical information under the Medicare+ Choice program guidelines (42 *U.S.C.* § 1395w-22[h], 2000). Under this statute the Medicare+Choice organization is required to establish procedures "to safeguard the privacy of any individually identifiable enrollee information." This provision does not ensure the information will be safe from legal discovery once sent to the federal government; however, it does help ensure that the Medicare+ Choice organization will not accidentally disclose sensitive information to a third party, thereby destroying any privilege or confidentiality that may exist from other sources. This provision applies only to Medicare+Choice organizations and does not give organizations any guidance for achieving confidentiality.

The Social Security Act goes one step further in protecting substance abuse and mental health records (42 *U.S.C.* § 290dd-2, 2000). It protects data relating to "the identity, diagnosis, prognosis, or treatment of any patient, which are maintained in connection with the performance of any program or activity relating to substance abuse education, prevention, training, treatment, rehabilitation, or research, which is conducted, regulated, or directly or indirectly assisted by any department or agency of the United States." This section specifically requires that no such information be used "to initiate or substantiate any criminal charges against a patient or to conduct any investigation of a patient." The information, however, may be released pursuant to a court order for good cause.

Under the Food, Drug, and Cosmetic Act, medical information regarding drug abuse prevention and control studies may be granted even stricter protection (21 *U.S.C.* § 872, 2000). This statute permits the attorney general to authorize persons engaged in such research to withhold the names and other identifying characteristics of research subjects: "Persons who obtain this authorization may not be compelled in any Federal, State or local civil, criminal, administrative, legislative or other proceeding to identify the subjects of research for which such authorization was obtained." This protection, however, does not apply when there is no authorization by the attorney general. A similar but broader protection is granted to research subjects under the Social Security Act. With the authorization of the secretary of HHS, researchers may withhold names and other identifying characteristics of any research subjects (42 *U.S.C.* § 241[d], 2000).

Researchers with authorization from the secretary cannot be compelled to divulge the names of research subjects or other identifying characteristics in any federal, state, or local civil or criminal proceeding.

Finally, the Veterans Health Administration protects confidential data relating to specific treatments or disorders (38 *U.S.C.* § 7332, 2000). Records containing the identity or treatment data of any patient relating to drug abuse, alcoholism, HIV infection, or sickle cell anemia are to be kept confidential. The section does allow disclosure of HIV status to the spouse or sexual partner of the patient under specific circumstances. Otherwise the statute provides protection except as authorized by court order. It also provides that no record may be used to initiate or substantiate any criminal charges against or to conduct any investigation of a patient or subject.

Health Insurance Portability and Accountability Act (HIPAA) Regulations. The HHS recently issued regulations intended to protect the privacy and confidentiality of medical records (45 *C.F.R.* Part 164, 2003). These regulations apply to *covered entities,* a term that includes health plans, health care clearinghouses, and health care providers who conduct certain financial and administrative transactions electronically. However, the regulations do not apply only to electronic transmissions. The final rules extend coverage to all medical record and other identifiable health information maintained or disclosed by a covered entity in any form, whether communicated electronically, on paper, or orally. The general rule is that the use or disclosure of *protected health information* (PHI) requires the patient's permission, except as permitted in the privacy regulations. Specifically, the rules permit use and disclosure in four circumstances. First, PHI can be released to the individual about whom the information was generated. Second, PHI can be released pursuant to a written consent for treatment, payment, or health care operations. Third, an individual may provide written consent to have his information released for any other purpose. Fourth, the rules establish certain exceptions under which PHI can be released, including emergency care situations and situations in which the care provider attempts but fails to obtain consent (45 *C.F.R.* §164.506[a]).

The rules also allow the covered entity the unlimited right to use and disclose *deidentified information,* that is, information that does not identify the individual or that the covered entity has no reasonable basis to believe can be used to identify the individual. A covered entity meets this standard either by making a statistical determination that the information is deidentified or by meeting a safe harbor provided in the rules.

Federal Peer Review Organization Regulations. *Peer review organization* (PRO) review of items or services provided to Medicare beneficiaries determines whether the provided services are reasonable and medically necessary, whether the care provided is complete and adequate, and whether the quality of services meets professionally recognized standards of health care. PRO review of Medicare services is governed by the Social Security Act and the regulations promulgated under that Act. Specifically, 42 *C.F.R.* Part 480 (2003) governs the acquisition, protection, and disclosure of PRO information. Generally, a PRO must disclose information in its possession to the identified patient if the patient requests the information in writing and all other patient and practitioner identifiers have been removed (42 *C.F.R.* § 480.132[a]). Before disclosing, the PRO must seek the advice of the practitioner who treated the patient regarding the appropriateness of direct disclosure (42 *C.F.R.* § 480.132[a][2]). The PRO need not disclose information to the patient if it believes that such a disclosure could harm the patient (42 *C.F.R.* § 480.132[c]). With its disclosure of confidential information to the patient, the PRO must include a written statement informing the recipient that the information may not be redisclosed (42 *C.F.R.* § 480.104[a][2]). A PRO may make a disclosure to the public of its interpretations and generalizations regarding the quality of health care, even where that disclosure identifies a particular institution (42 *C.F.R.* § 480.141). Such disclosures are, however, governed by the requirements of 42 *C.F.R.* §§ 480.104 and 480.105. These regulations provide that the PRO must disclose the information only in the format in which the PRO uses the information and that the PRO must give the institution thirty days notice of its intent to disclose the information.

Protection Offered by Proposed Legislation. In 2002, a bill was introduced into Congress that directly addressed medical error management and reduction. Whether or not this bill ultimately passes, it signals the direction in which Congress may be headed. The Patient Safety Improvement Act of 2002 (HR 4889) would designate patient safety data as privileged and confidential. That designation would apply to information, such as medical records and other primary health care information, that is collected and developed for the purpose of improving patient safety and health care quality and reported to a patient safety organization such as a peer review organization or a quality committee. This privilege, however, would not apply to information merely by reason of its inclusion in reported patient safety data. Information available from sources other than a report made to a patient safety organization may be discovered or admitted in civil or administrative proceedings if discoverable under state law. Furthermore this privilege would not apply to records of a patient's medical diagnosis and treatment, data disclosed to the FDA, or disclosures of non-identifiable patient safety data by the patient safety organization to a patient safety database.

Common Law Protection

The extent to which physician-patient and psychotherapist-patient privileges exist have been determined largely by the courts.

Physician-Patient Privilege. The federal courts do not recognize a physician-patient privilege, although confidentiality between a patient and a physician has in some cases been deemed a constitutionally protected zone of privacy. The U.S. Supreme Court has used an intermediate scrutiny test to balance the "public and private interests" in the confidentiality of these communications (*Whalen* v. *Roe,* 1977). The Court did not, however, go so far as to establish an absolute privacy interest in confidential medical records information. In fact there is a hearsay exception to the Federal Rules of Evidence for medical records.

The issue in *Whalen* was whether the state of New York could record, in a centralized computer file, the names and addresses of all persons who obtained, pursuant to a legal prescription, certain drugs, including cocaine, methadone, and amphetamines, for which there is both a lawful and an unlawful market. Although the appellees offered some evidence that tended to show that persons in need of treatment with these drugs will sometimes decline such treatment out of fear of being labeled a drug addict, the Court found that the public benefit outweighed any burden on privacy. It is important that in this case, public disclosure of the identity of patients was expressly prohibited by the statute at issue, the New York State Controlled Substance Act of 1972 (N.Y. Pub. Health Law § 3300 *et seq.,* 1976). The Court therefore found that it did not need to address "any question which might be presented by the unwarranted disclosure of accumulated personal data—whether intentional or unintentional." Lower courts have applied this same balancing test in deciding to permit disclosure of medical records. For example, in *In re Krynecki* (1993) the court of appeals ordered disclosure. In *Krynecki* a physician objected to a grand jury subpoena for medical records of 120 patients on the grounds that releasing the records would violate patients' privacy. The court recognized the potential burden on privacy but did not agree such a burden was present in this case. The court made its determination on the premise that the "confidentiality of the grand jury process sufficiently offset that concern."

Psychotherapist-Patient Privilege. Although there is no physician-patient privilege recognized at common law, in *Jaffee* v. *Redmond* (1996) the Supreme Court recognized a psychotherapist-patient privilege. In *Jaffee,* the petitioner requested notes from the respondent's psychotherapist sessions during discovery. The respondent, a former police officer who had shot the petitioner's decedent, in the line of duty, refused to disclose the notes. The issue for the Court was whether it is appropriate for federal courts to recognize a "psychotherapist privilege" under Rule 501 of the Federal Rules of Evidence. The Court held that a psychotherapist privilege should apply to prevent disclosure of the notes in this case. The Court reasoned that like the "spousal and attorney-client privileges, the psychotherapist-patient privilege is 'rooted in the imperative need for confidence and trust.'" The Court differentiated treatment by a physician that often is accomplished on the basis of a purely physical examination and psychotherapy that depends on the patient's being able to "make a frank and complete disclosure of facts, emotions, memories and fears." The Court went even further, rejecting the balancing component used by lower courts, because making confidentiality contingent on whether a trial judge felt the privacy interest outweighed the public interest effectively eviscerated the privilege. In other words, the participants to the confidential conversation "must be able to predict with some degree of certainty whether particular discussions will be protected."

Conclusion

There are grounds for concern that sharing medical error data with the government or an accrediting agency will waive any privilege that may have previously protected that information from discovery. As described in the chapter the states and the federal government have various ways in which to protect medical error data. Judging from the actions of some states and the federal government, legislatures are finding it increasingly important to protect such data to promote reporting and to foster improved patient safety.

References

Amente v. Newman, 653 So. 2d 1030 (Fla. 1995).

American Jurisprudence, s.v. "Second Witnesses," vol. 81, § 474, 2004.

Babcock v. Bridgeport Hospital, 742 A.2d 822 (Conn. 1999).

Beck v. Bluestein, 476 A.2d 842 (N.J. Sup. Ct. App. Div. 1984).

Berger v. Lutheran General Hospital, 2001 Ill. LEXIS 1423 (Oct. 18, 2001).

Centers for Disease Control and Prevention. "About NNIS."
    [http://www.cdc.gov/ncidod/hip/NNIS/@nnis.htm]. Sept. 2003.

Chicago Trust Co. v. Cook County Hospital, 698 N.E.2d 641 (Ill. App. Ct. 1998).

Cochran v. St. Paul Fire and Marine Insurance Co., 909 F. Supp. 641 (W.D. Ark. 1995).

Community Hospital of Indianapolis v. Medtronic, 594 N.E.2d 448 (Ind. App. 1st Dist. 1992).

Corrigan v. Methodist Hospital, 885 F. Supp. 127 (E.D. Pa. 1995).

Doe v. Stephens, 851 F.2d 1457 (D.C. Cir. 1988).

Dorris v. *Detroit Osteopathic Hospital Corp.,* 594 N.W.2d 455 (Mich. 1999).

Ekstrom v. *Temple,* 553 N.E.2d 424 (2d Dist. 1990).

Fox v. *Kramer,* 70 Cal. App. 4th 177, 82 Cal. Rptr. 2d 513 (6th Dist. 1999).

Henkel, J. "MedWatch: FDA's 'Heads Up' on Medical Product Safety." *FDA Consumer,* 1998, *32*(6), 10–12, 15.

In re Krynecki, 1993 U.S. App. LEXIS 21759 (7th Cir.), *cert. denied,* 510 U.S. 1118 (1994).

Jaffee v. *Redmond,* 518 U.S. 1 (1996).

John C. Lincoln Hospital and Health Center v. *Superior Court,* 768 P.2d 188 (Ariz. Ct. App. 1989).

Kappas v. *Chestnut Lodge, Inc.,* 709 F.2d 878 (4th Cir. 1983).

Kimberlin v. *U.S. Department of Justice,* 788 F.2d 434 (7th Cir. 1986).

Kutner v. *Davenport,* 360 S.E.2d 586 (Ga. 1987).

McMaster v. *Board of Psychology Examiners,* 509 N.W. 2d 754, 757 (Iowa 1993), *cert. denied,* 114 S. Ct. 2165 (1994).

Mulder v. *VanKersen,* 637 N.E.2d 1335 (Ind. Ct. App. 1994).

Nielson v. *Bryson,* 477 P.2d 714 (Ore. 1970).

Painting Industry of Hawaii v. *Department of the Air Force,* 26 F.3d 1479 (9th Cir. 1994).

Parton v. *U.S. Department of Justice,* 727 F.2d 774 (8th Cir. 1984).

Payne v. *Howard,* 75 F.R.D. 465 (D. D.C. 1977).

Reproductive Services v. *Walker,* 439 U.S. 1307, 1308–1309 (1978).

Roberts v. *Department of Health and Human Services,* 1988 U.S. Dist. LEXIS 10162 (E.D. Pa).

Robinson, A. R., and others. "Physician and Public Opinions on Quality of Health Care and the Problem of Medical Errors." *Archives of Internal Medicine,* Oct. 28, 2002, *162,* 2186–2190.

Rosenthal, J., Riley, T., and Booth, M. *State Reporting of Medical Errors and Adverse Events: Results of a 50-State Survey.* Portland, Maine: National Academy for State Health Policy, 2000.

Rothschild, J. M., and others. "Analysis of Medication-Related Malpractice Claims: Causes, Preventability, and Costs." *Archives of Internal Medicine,* Nov. 25, 2002, *162,* 2414–2420.

Sakosko v. *Memorial Hospital,* 167 Ill. App. 3d 842, 118 Ill. Dec. 818, 522 N.E.2d 273 (5th Dist. 1988).

Santa Rosa Memorial Hospital v. *Superior Court,* 174 Cal. App. 3d 711, 220 Cal. Rptr. 236 (1st Dist. 1985).

State ex rel. St. John's Mercy Medical Center v. *Hoester,* 708 S.W.2d 796 (E.D. Mo. Ct. App. 1986).

Suwannee County Hospital Corporation v. *Meeks,* 472 So.2d 1305 (Fla. Dist. Ct. App. 1985).

United States v. *AT&T,* 642 F.2d 1285, 1299 (D.C. Cir. 1980).

U.S. Department of Justice v. *Tax Analysts,* 492 U.S. 136 (1988).

U.S. Department of State v. *Ray,* 502 U.S. 164 (1991).

University of Texas Health Science Center v. *Jordan,* 686 S.W.2d 652 (Tex. App. 1985).

Wall v. *Ohio Permanente Medical Group, Inc.,* 695 N.E.2d 1233 (Ohio Ct. App. 1997).

Whalen v. *Roe,* 429 U.S. 589 (1977).

Wigmore, J. H. *Evidence in Trials at Common Law.* Vol. 8 (rev. by J. T. McNaughton). Boston: Little, Brown, 1961.

Williams v. *Roosevelt Hospital,* 66 N.Y.2d 391, 395 (N.Y. 1985).

Wright, C. A., Miller, A. R., and others. *Federal Practice and Procedure: Civil 2d* § 2035. St. Paul, Minn.: West, 1998.

York v. *American Medical Systems,* 1998 U.S. App. LEXIS 30105 (6th Cir. 1998).

CHAPTER TWELVE

MANAGING PATIENT SAFETY COMPLIANCE WITH HEALTH PROFESSIONALS

Mark A. Kadzielski
Christina W. Giles

Dealing with quality issues as systems problems that require improvement is often a difficult balancing act. Typically, every person involved in the specific health care setting is a responsible team member, but when substandard performance is noted on the part of one or more individuals, it becomes very difficult to handle in a positive way. The fact that quality is everyone's number one job, whether he or she is toiling in housekeeping, materials management, or critical care nursing, is an important concept in the health care setting. However, even though this general focus appropriately shapes the discussion, and has become the mantra of quality professionals and health care leaders, it is definitely not the only focus.

Employment and Disciplinary Issues

To generalize quality as a systems issue is not to deny that in individual circumstances individual health care professionals may perform below acceptable standards. Steps must be taken to deal with the individual involved in the substandard performance in order to change the quality outcome, whether or not the performance results in injury to patients. If action is not taken, the rest of the health care team will be doing little more than shifting resources and covering up for the poor performance of a colleague. This scenario occurs more often than we realize, but its dynamics must be understood and addressed by those in health care who are serious about making inroads into the difficult quality issues that exist.

Temporary Suspension and Other Options

When individuals are identified as potentially involved in the performance of substandard care, regardless of outcome, the first step is to consider the alternatives from an employment and staff privileges point of view. When such problem performers are identified initially, many health institutions feel trapped between two extreme but natural courses of action: to do nothing or to take immediate drastic measures, such as termination or suspension without pay for employees or some type of corrective action for licensed independent practitioners who have been granted privileges. These alternatives create many legal risks and may do very little to provide an understanding of the context of the error or of the ultimate methods for avoiding similar errors in the future. Certainly, the suspended or terminated health care professional will have very little incentive to cooperate in subsequent investigations while being economically penalized. By taking such summary action the institution may indeed be depriving itself of an important source of information for identifying the factual and environmental background of the incident. The fact that terminated or suspended health care professionals also have legal rights and are willing to enforce these rights in litigation against the provider makes this situation even more unpredictable.

It is important that health care providers understand that their options are not limited to these two extremes, and that they can adopt many measures short of outright termination or suspension without pay. These measures are not only less onerous on the individual but also create an entirely different atmosphere in which to conduct an investigation and to enlist the assistance of the individual health care providers involved. Among these options are *monitoring*—another professional checks on or observes the performance of the health professional suspected of poor performance; *job reassignment*—the health professional works in an area apart from the service where the incident occurred; and *temporary suspension* with pay for a designed limited period of time while an investigation that includes the involved professional takes place. Obviously, no one of these options is appropriate in all situations, but they all need to be considered as alternatives to the status quo, where inertia in the face of quality problems has for too long been the acceptable response. If we are to address patient safety responsibly, the choice is not all or nothing. Health care providers must take some action because taking no action is unacceptable and may well lead to disastrous results in the future.

The health care professional who may feel singled out unfairly for the unwarranted attention of monitoring or job reassignment cannot claim any economic harm from such action. If the investigation reveals that there is no reason to continue such actions, the professional can return to his or her position and continue to practice as before. Such monitoring or reassignment may also have the salutary effect of refocusing the professional on the basics of his or her job and the quality of his or her performance. Temporary suspension, however, must be handled more delicately, because the professional is going to be removed from the workplace for a period of time and the psychological ramifications from that process may be debilitating. The best way to handle this option is to conduct a detailed interview with the professional prior to the actual suspension and to make it clear that the suspension is temporary and is with full pay. Regular follow-ups by telephone with the professional should occur every few days or at least weekly to provide updates on the general status of the investigation and the prospects of returning to work.

Employee Assistance Programs

Additional consideration should be given to the fact that the health care professional may also be in need of health care services to resolve the issue. In today's managed care environment, where patient care encounters are measured and payment is capitated, there is great pressure on all health care professionals to do more with less. Maximizing revenues in health care means seeing as many patients as possible in as short amount of time as possible, doing more procedures quicker, and performing more tests and processing more physician orders. Harried professionals tend to make more mistakes. Caregiver *burnout* is a common phenomenon in health care.

In this context, patient safety investigations may result in the recognition that caregivers involved in quality issues may themselves benefit from therapy, counseling, or other programs offered by the institutional *employee assistance program* (EAP). Before referring such caregivers to the EAP, however, it must be decided whether the EAP will be able to provide the level of intervention needed for the health care professional to continue in his or her current position. If the investigation process concludes that the health care professional would greatly benefit from some relaxation or stress reduction or other ongoing counseling, the EAP may be an appropriate referral for that individual. If the issues run deeper, the EAP is probably not the only resource that should be considered. For example, if it is determined that the individual has a chemical dependency that impairs job performance, time off to attend an inpatient treatment and recovery program might be considered, and it might not be appropriate to use the EAP except for purposes of aftercare, such as monitoring ongoing participation in Alcoholics Anonymous (AA) or Narcotics Anonymous (NA) meetings. In any event the judicious use of the resources afforded by the health care institution's own EAP should be a consideration in the process of dealing with the caregiver involved in quality problems.

Disciplinary Actions

Disciplinary actions against health care professionals involved in quality problems are also varied, and a number of alternatives are available to health care institutions. Summary actions, such as the temporary suspension with pay already discussed, are the first level of disciplinary action. In general, summary suspension for an indefinite period without pay and immediate termination are remedies that should be used only in the most egregious cases. Criminal activity, for example, may well warrant such actions. However, less drastic disciplinary actions are much more commonplace in dealing with perceived quality issues. Actions such as demotion, reduction in benefits, or a salary freeze for confirmed quality problems may well have a more persuasive effect on the individual health care professional because they give the person an opportunity to keep his or her job and an incentive to restore the benefits lost through exemplary work in the future. Ongoing counseling and job retraining may be an important concurrent aspect of such disciplinary actions. Indeed, the disciplinary actions may be imposed for only a limited period, pending the outcome of retraining or remedial coursework.

Although the measures just described may be effective for employees of health institutions, licensed physicians, dentists, podiatrists, and members of other allied health professions are often not considered employees for various reasons, such as the corporate practice of medicine doctrine. This doctrine prohibits the *lay practice* of a profession and has been held to prevent the direct employment of such professionals by health care institutions. In such cases these individuals are subject not to the disciplinary actions of the institution's human resource policies and procedures but rather to the provisions of those documents under which they are granted the right to practice in the institution, under the rubric of professional staff membership and clinical privileges. Thus the disciplinary actions applicable to such professionals are contained in the governing documents of the professional staff, namely its bylaws and rules and regulations.

Bylaws and rules and regulations for professional staff almost uniformly provide for various types or levels of disciplinary action against staff members and others who are permitted to practice in the health care institution. These actions include, but are not limited to, revocation, suspension, limitation, modification, and significant proctoring of a health care professional's privileges to attend patients. Termination, suspension, or demotion in membership status are additional disciplinary actions that may be taken.

Many if not most of these proposed actions, under the terms of bylaws, will afford the practitioner rights to hearings and appeals before the discipline becomes final. This is due to various legal decisions that health professionals have important *property rights* in the privileges granted to them. Although a plethora of cases have been decided on this issue, it is significant that employees generally are provided fewer opportunities for hearings prior to the imposition of disciplinary action (Kadzielski, 2002). One exception to this situation lies in the unionized health care workplace, where the labor union member has a right to grieve a job action taken by the employer and may have a right to have it arbitrated or resolved in some neutral setting prior to its being imposed.

Unions, Collective Agreements, and Patient Safety Compliance

In the unionized environment health care workers are protected by the collective bargaining agreements between their unions and the health care institutions that employ them. Such agreements often provide for grievance procedures and for other collective processes when the discipline of an individual union member is contemplated. Although health care unions have spoken out forcefully on the issue of patient safety and have acted to protect the interests of patients by arguing for better staffing ratios and more qualified personnel, the admitted primary self-interest of the union is to protect its members and its members' jobs. Where it has been established that disciplinary action is appropriate against an employee who is a union member, the union should be put on notice of this possibility as early as possible. Involving the union representative, shop steward, or other superior in the initial quality issue investigation will go a long way toward ensuring buy-in on the ultimate result, especially if it involves disciplining a union member.

The Credentialing Process as a Patient Safety Tool

Most laypeople are unaware of the credentialing process that takes place in health care institutions. Even health care workers, unless they have personally experienced the credentialing process, are not aware of what it entails and how it truly affects patients. It consists of four major steps: (1) information collection, (2) information verification, (3) assessment of information and recommendation, and (4) the granting of authority to practice (National Association Medical Staff Services, 2003, § 1). Anyone who has been involved in the credentialing process is well aware of the fact that this process is performed for many reasons, but the first and foremost reason is patient safety. This process assists a hospital's medical staff, administration, and board of trustees to make responsible and objective judgments and to assign authority to practice to appropriately trained, experienced, and competent practitioners.

Many Web sites have been developed to provide the consumer with information about physicians and other health care practitioners—their training, experience, and in some cases clinical practice—and to allow consumers to compare practitioners. Only experienced and trained credentialing personnel are knowledgeable about the information sites and sources accepted by accrediting agencies such as the Joint Commission on Accreditation of Healthcare Organizations (JCAHO), National Committee for Quality Assurance (NCQA), Accreditation Association for Ambulatory Health Care (AAAHC), and URAC. By using acceptable primary or designated equivalent sources in the credentialing process, the health care organization ensures compliance with accrediting body requirements and also collects thorough and appropriate information on which the relevant medical staff leaders and committees and board of trustee members can base their decisions.

The credentialing process typically begins by collecting information from the physician or other health care practitioner by means of an application that requests all the information the organization requires. Copies of certain documents such as the medical license, DEA (Drug Enforcement Administration) certificate, and specialty board certificate are also often requested. When an incomplete application is received or when gaps of time are identified in the applicant's training or work experience, then no further assessment of the applicant is performed until all the missing information is supplied or the gaps are explained. The trained credentialing professional is then able to begin the verification process, which includes verifying the information supplied by the applicant with acceptable primary sources or, if allowed, designated equivalent or secondary sources. All the documentation is organized and placed in a file that is then reviewed by multiple designated medical staff leaders and committees. If all individuals and committees concur with the positive recommendations of the initial individual's or committee's recommendation, then the applicant is granted membership or privileges, or both, on the medical or professional staff. The most important part of this process is obtaining sufficient information—via peers of the applicant, previous supervisors or colleagues, and training institutions—in the form of supportive commentary on the applicant's clinical judgment, medical knowledge, clinical skills, human interaction skills, professionalism, provision of care, and moral and ethical behavior. The initial appointment period is typically for one year, during which time the appointee is observed, assessed, and provided with feedback on his or her clinical work and observation of and compliance with the institution's rules, regulations, policies, and procedures. Once the appointee has fulfilled the provisional year requirements satisfactorily, then he or she is assessed every two years for reappointment to the staff, unless the provisional period has been extended for an additional year to continue the observation and assessment. Every two years the process is performed again: information collection, verification, assessment, and recommendation and granting of authority to practice. Individuals and committees have multiple opportunities to provide input to the assessment of new appointees and long-term members. The end result of this process should be an assurance that only competent, knowledgeable practitioners practice at the health care institution, thus protecting the patient from being treated by an incompetent or impaired practitioner.

Typically, such informational items as licensure; completion of accredited, appropriate training; specialty board certification; malpractice history; and history of sanctions are collected and used in the credentialing process. Every one of the fifty states has a medical licensing board that collects information from the physician and verifies that information prior to granting a medical license. The states vary, however, in their specific requirements for licensure, ranging from requiring the completion of four years of medical school and one year of postgraduate training to the completion of a three-year residency program. Specialty board certification, sponsored by the American Board of Medical Specialties, the American Osteopathic Association, the American Podiatric Association, and the American Dental Association (the most widely accepted specialty boards in most U.S. hospitals), requires completion of at least a three-year postgraduate, accredited training program and, for some special qualification certificates, additional years of training. The two elements of licensure and specialty certification have become the minimum standard for most health care organizations. Obviously, no one can practice medicine without a state license. However, because licensure requires a minimal amount of education and training and because many licensing boards have been lax and slow in disciplining physicians who have been reported (Larry, Wolfe, and Lurie, 2000), having a current license in good standing has become a legal requirement rather than a measurement of quality (Ginsburg and Moy, 1992). Many managed care organizations and hospitals have established a minimum requirement of specialty board certification prior to considering an applicant for membership, privileges, or participation as a provider. Some information collected during the credentialing process is required by the accrediting organization; other information is identified by the health care organization. All items of information are pieces of the credentialing pie and should be reviewed in the aggregate rather than separately.

Occasionally, quality problems arise with practitioners who have been reviewed and assessed in the credentialing process. Patient safety is always of utmost concern; however, built into the process are some protections for health care practitioners who have been granted privileges and who are now experiencing difficulties, whether physical, mental, or emotional. The goal of the medical staff is to assist the practitioner in resolving whatever problem has arisen and to identify opportunities for the practitioner to obtain assistance, complete a rehabilitation or treatment program, and reenter practice and treat patients safely. Since 2001, JCAHO has introduced many new medical staff standards, one of which addresses having a nonpunitive approach to physician health that is separate from the disciplinary process. JCAHO's medical staff standards (JCAHO, 2004a, Standard MS.4.80) state that a physician health program has to involve

1. Education of [licensed independent practitioners] LIPs and other hospital staff about illness and impairment recognition issues specific to LIPs (at-risk criteria).
2. Self referral by an LIP.
3. Referral by others and creation of confidentiality of informants.
4. Referral of the affected LIP to appropriate professional internal or external resources for evaluation, diagnosis, and treatment of the condition or concern.
5. Maintenance of confidentiality of the LIP seeking referral or referred for assistance, except as limited by law or ethical obligation or when the health and safety of a patient is threatened.
6. Evaluation of the credibility of a complaint, allegation, or concern.
7. Monitoring the affected LIP and the safety of patients until the rehabilitation or any disciplinary process is complete and periodically thereafter, if required.
8. Reporting to the organized medical staff leadership instances in which an LIP is providing unsafe treatment.

Most state medical societies have established successful physician health programs that assist in assessing the physician to determine the extent of the impairment (physical, mental, or emotional) and to prepare a plan for treatment or rehabilitation. These programs typically work in conjunction with licensing boards under an agreement that if the physician agrees to the proposed treatment or rehabilitation plan, she or he will not be reported to the licensing board; however, if she or he does not comply with or complete the treatment or program, then a report will be submitted to the licensing board and the physician will risk disciplinary action from the licensing board as well as a report to the National Practitioner Data Bank. Referral to a medical society program is not always available to other health care practitioners; thus the health care organization is often responsible for overseeing treatment or rehabilitation for nonphysician independent health care providers.

There are many programs and organizations that have begun to influence how health care practitioners are handled when problems have been identified and that thus affect patient safety. One such program, founded in 1990 in Aurora, Colorado, is the Center for Personalized Education for Physicians (CPEP, 2004). CPEP is modeled on a three-step process of assessment; development of an educational intervention; and evaluation focusing on the physician-participant's medical knowledge, clinical reasoning, communication skills, and patient care documentation. Educational objectives are developed based on the assessment findings and a focused, intensive, and personalized educational program is outlined for the participant. CPEP assists the participant with arranging the activities necessary to achieve the educational program objectives and monitors his or her progress. Follow-up evaluations are conducted to document fulfillment of educational objectives and findings are reported to the participant and to relevant organizations when appropriate. This program is available to physicians who are seeking assistance in addressing state licensing boards, peer review organizations (PROs), or hospital patient care concerns; who are planning a career transition or returning to clinical practice after an absence; who are recovering from a disabling accident or illness; or who are seeking to update their clinical knowledge and technical skills.

A second group, the Leapfrog Group, with a membership of more than 150 public and private organizations that provide health care benefits, works with medical experts throughout the United States to identify problems and propose solutions that it believes will improve hospital systems at risk of breaking down and harming patients. Representing more than thirty-one million health care consumers in all fifty states, Leapfrog provides important information and solutions for consumers and health care providers and has so far presented three initiatives to improve patient safety (Leapfrog Group, 2004). One of these initiatives involves intensive care unit (ICU) physician staffing. The Leapfrog Group's recommendation is that a physician certified or qualified for certification in critical care medicine should manage hospital ICUs. A majority of the smaller community hospitals in the United States have *open ICUs*—they allow any member of the medical staff who has had some training in caring for critically ill patients to admit and manage the ICU patient. In comparison to all other types of board-certified specialists, there are very few board-certified critical care specialists. The American Boards of Anesthesiology, Internal Medicine, Obstetrics and Gynecology, Pediatrics, and General Surgery all offer subspecialty certificates in critical care; yet according to the American Board of Medical Specialties (ABMS, 2004), the following numbers of individuals received a subspecialty certificate in critical care from 1994 to 2003: anesthesiology, 476; internal medicine, 3,514; obstetrics and gynecology, 3; pediatrics, 688; general surgery, 752. The total number of critical care subspecialty certificates awarded from 1994 to 2003 was 5,433; the total number of general certificates awarded in those same specialties during the same time period was 132,885. The credentialing process will identify those who have achieved critical care subspecialty certification and that information can be verified by contacting the ABMS, the individual specialty board, or a designated equivalent source. Most certifications now have a time limit; once certification expires, unless the physician has taken another exam, that certification is no longer valid. The American Osteopathic Association (2004) also has general certifications, certification of special qualifications, and certification of added qualifications. In the last category, only the AOA Boards of Anesthesiology, Internal Medicine, and Surgery provide a certificate in added qualifications for critical care.

According to Leapfrog's "ICU Physician Staffing Factsheet," mortality rates are significantly lower in hospitals with closed ICUs managed exclusively by board-certified critical care specialists, or *intensivists*. A study conducted by Peter Pronovost, an intensivist at Johns Hopkins Medical Institutions, found that high-intensity ICU staffing (where intensivists manage or comanage all patients), as opposed to low-intensity ICU staffing (where intensivists manage or comanage some or none of the patients), is associated with a 30 percent reduction in hospital mortality and a 40 percent reduction in ICU mortality (Leapfrog Group, 2003). However, the reality is that the number of certified critical care specialists is insufficient to support all the ICUs in the United States; thus the next best approach would be for hospitals to develop strict criteria for granting critical care privileges, rather than granting privileges to physicians who cannot document recent critical care experience with satisfactory outcomes. The privileging process in most hospitals is currently not sophisticated enough to collect and analyze such documentation prior to granting privileges to manage ICU patients; but many hospitals are well on the way to requiring the necessary documentation for better assessment of ICU skills and knowledge. JCAHO recently has proposed to join forces with the Leapfrog Group to identify other recommendations concerning patient safety in all hospital ICUs in light of the insufficient numbers of physicians trained in this subspecialty. In addition, JCAHO has established seven national patient safety goals for 2004. Each goal includes no more than two succinct, evidence- or expert-based recommendations. These goals are addressed in hospital accreditation surveys—all hospitals must have implemented mechanisms for compliance with or acceptable alternatives to the following goals (JCAHO, 2004b):

1. Improve the accuracy of patient identification.
2. Improve the effectiveness of communication among caregivers.
3. Improve the safety of using high-alert medications.

4. Reduce wrong-site, wrong-patient, wrong-procedure surgery.
5. Improve the safety of using infusion pumps.
6. Improve the effectiveness of clinical alarm systems.
7. Reduce the risk of health care–acquired infections.

The 2005 Hospital Patient Safety Goals differ on two goals. Goal 5 will be, "Accurately and completely reconcile medications across the continuum of care," and Goal 6 will be, "Reduce the risk of patient harm resulting from falls."

Another program that should have an effect on patient safety is the Practitioner Remediation and Enhancement Partnership (PREP). The Citizen Advocacy Center has contracted "with the Health Resources and Services Administration (HRSA) to set up pilot projects around the country involving hospitals and boards of medicine and nursing in partnerships to enhance health care quality by improving information sharing and other forms of cooperation between health care providers and regulators" (Citizen Advocacy Center, 2004). This project will "institutionalize information sharing" between hospitals and licensing boards when one or the other of these entities identifies a practitioner whose performance is not up to an acceptable standard of quality and it will recommend remedial actions, such as targeted education, to upgrade the practitioner's competence or impose practice restrictions or specialized supervision and monitoring (4PatientSafety.net, 2002). The organizations participating in this project include state medical and osteopathic licensing boards and nursing licensure boards. "It is the goal of this project to enhance communication among hospitals, licensing boards, and other relevant agencies and to move from a disciplinary approach to one of education and learning while ensuring protection of patients." As of April 2002, the following boards of medicine had voted to participate: California, Minnesota, Missouri, North Carolina, Oregon, and Rhode Island. The following boards of nursing have voted to participate: Colorado, Maryland, Nebraska, North Carolina, Oregon, and South Carolina and also the West Virginia Board of Examiners for Licensed Practical Nurses. The PREP programs are operational in boards in three states: the North Carolina Board of Nursing, the West Virginia Board of Examiners for Licensed Practical Nurses, and the California Medical Board (Citizen Advocacy Center, 2002).

Physician *report cards* are becoming increasingly popular and are beginning to be used by various managed care organizations across the country. Tufts Health Plan, based in Boston, has announced a Physician Group Quality Profile Report that is available to current and prospective patients to guide them in making informed choices when selecting where to seek care and to assist providers in continuing to improve care. Tufts claims to be the first managed care organization on the East Coast to release such information. "The report compares more than one hundred physician groups to national benchmarks in six areas." Members are asked about the following measures: satisfaction with the primary care doctor, access to specialty care, wait time for appointments, outcome of care, personal interest in you. Preventive care measures include the following: rate of examination of diabetic patients' eyes, rate of breast cancer screening, and rate of cervical cancer screening. Pediatric preventive measures include well-child visits and adolescent well-care visits. Tufts representatives state that "reporting on a larger group of physicians with more eligible members allows for a better reflection of the services provided. It also helps avoid statistical aberrations caused by using the data from small groups of patients and helps maintain statistical validity" (Tufts Health Plan, 2004).

A weakness in the current system is the lack of measurement, assessment, and development of supportive mechanisms for practitioners other than physicians. The PREP program will be available to nurses, but a multitude of other health care practitioners—physician assistants, physical therapists, advanced practice nurses, chiropractors, and psychologists, to name a few—may not have similar programs to turn to for assistance. When a problem with any of these practitioners is identified, much less assistance and rehabilitation seems to be available. The onus is on the practitioner and the health care organization to provide oversight of practice and to maintain patient safety by identifying problems and arranging for referrals for appropriate treatment.

Another weak spot in the system involves physicians in training. *Interns, residents, and fellows* are physicians in training. Typically, these individuals are not credentialed in the same way that licensed independent practitioners are. There is some checking of backgrounds but horror stories such as the activities of Dr. Swango ("Dr. Death"), still rear their ugly heads (Stewart, 1999). JCAHO has instituted a new standard and revised other standards (effective January 1, 2002, 2003, and 2004) concerning the supervision of residents. The medical staff of a hospital are responsible for the quality of the professional services provided by licensed independent practitioners and by participants in a professional graduate education program. JCAHO Standard MS.2.30 addresses graduate education programs. EP 2 states: "Written descriptions of the roles, responsibilities, and patient care activities of participants in professional graduate education programs are provided to the organized medical staff and hospital staff." "The organized medical staff must have a defined process for supervision, by an LIP with appropriate clinical privileges, of each participant in the program in carrying out his or her patient care responsibilities. The descriptions must include identification of mechanisms by which the supervisor(s) and graduate education program director make decisions about each participant's progressive involvement and independence in specific patient care activities" (JCAHO, 2004a). Typically residents and fellows are treated as employees rather than as medical staff members. Thus, if a problem arises with a physician in training, the issue is addressed through human resource policies and procedures. If there is a health or addiction problem, the individual is referred to the employee assistance program. More than likely, if the resident or fellow is not compliant with the proposed treatment or program, he or she will not be allowed to continue in the program. Unfortunately, many programs are not truthful about the reasons for a physician's departure. Thus it is very likely that the physician in training might well be accepted to participate in another training program with few questions asked about what happened at the original program.

The credentialing process is an important tool used by many types of health care organizations to protect the patient. The reason for using the process is to ensure that each applicant is who she or he says she or he is, and is capable of providing the services requested. A great deal of detective work is done prior to allowing a new practitioner to practice in an institution. Weaknesses in the process are often revealed when a long-time medical staff member begins to experience mental, physical, or emotional difficulties. Although many hospitals have initiated well-developed physician well-being programs, there is still a reluctance to "turn in" and monitor a colleague. Patient safety is the reason that spurs medical staff into action, but oftentimes the action could have been taken sooner. The review process for accepting a physician into a training program needs to become more stringent; additional information needs to be collected and assessed. These steps should be more like the credentialing process used prior to the acceptance of a new resident into a program. If there is a problem, better documentation and communication concerning the action taken must be initiated. If the resident is asked to leave, any future programs that she or he applies to must be supplied with relevant information about the action that took place and the reasons for it. Corporate accountability and liability exist for all health care organizations that provide health services and allow practitioners—physicians and nonphysicians—to provide those services to patients. If the organized medical staff fail to perform their duty in terms of assessing and recommending applicants for staff membership or privileges, then it is incumbent upon the board of trustees of each institution to become involved. They must ensure that the credentialing process is sufficiently thorough to identify applicants for appointment, reappointment, or privileges who have key issues and that there are written policies to assist the medical staff in handling those situations. They also need to ensure that basic requirements placed upon prospective employees, such as specific disease testing or criminal background checks, are applied equally to prospective medical and professional staff members—there should be no difference in the prerequisites for prospective employees and prospective medical or professional staff members when it comes to protecting the safety of the patient.

The Difference Between Corrective Action and Blame

The recent Institute of Medicine (IOM) reports *To Err Is Human* and *Crossing the Quality Chasm* both make the point that in order for America's health care system to survive, organizations have to move away from blaming individuals for errors and move toward a team approach to preventing error, where everyone is involved in collecting and analyzing useful data to determine problems; formulate solutions; and test, implement, and measure outcomes to improve patient safety. Today's organizations must move from asking, "Whose fault was this?" to asking, "Why did this error occur and what can we do to prevent it from occurring again?" A proactive approach is more productive than a reactive approach. In other words, a culture of safety must be established in which people are able to report adverse events and close calls without fear of punishment (Kohn, Corrigan, and Donaldson, 2000; IOM, 2001; Kadzielski and Martin, 2001, 2002).

In reality, most health care institutions have continued to look for the bad apple. Taking action against that bad apple has resulted in some practitioners' being fired or having privileges suspended, revoked, or altered in some way. Many of the sentinel events or bad outcomes noted by health care institutions are in fact the result of a series of problems within a specific process or multiple processes involved in patient care. However, sometimes the fault does lie with an individual who cannot be retrained or rehabilitated. In the case of an employee, the human resource policy dictates how that employee will be handled. In most instances, a collegial, educative approach is used initially, a plan of correction is outlined, and ongoing evaluation takes place to ensure that the change(s) are made in practice. If the situation involves a licensed independent practitioner who has been granted privileges in a hospital, then the same collegial approach is usually taken; the practitioner is allowed an opportunity to change his or her "ways"—to obtain additional education or to perform in a monitored situation for a period of time. In a managed care setting, the health care organization will often require a corrective action plan and afford the practitioner an opportunity to remedy the problem prior to removing him or her from the provider panel. Only when no change in behavior or practice is noted, after repeated attempts to assist the individual, will the typical medical staff begin the corrective action process outlined in the medical staff bylaws or policies and procedures. *Corrective action* is just what it says, an action taken to make a correction. This process may result in a formal disciplinary action taken against the medical staff member's privileges. This action may be reportable to the state licensing board and the National Practitioner Data Bank.

Conclusion

It is a proven fact that when individuals are feeling secure in their work environment and are informed that their practice or patient care is different from that of the majority of similar practitioners or that their cases have been reviewed and alternative approaches need to be taken, they will most likely change, remedying the problem. The organization is accountable for having a performance improvement process that works and that identifies system problems and distinguishes them from individual practitioner problems. This in turn will lead to a positive process when an individual does have to be approached and changes in behavior or practice must be requested.

References

American Board of Medical Specialties. *The ABMS Annual Report and Reference Handbook.* Evanston, Ill.: American Board of Medical Specialties, 2004.

American Osteopathic Association. [http://www.aoa-net.org/certification/jurisgeneral.htm]. 2004.

Center for Personalized Education for Physicians. [http://www.cpepdoc.org]. 2004.

Centers for Medicare & Medicaid Services, Center for Medicaid and State Operations/ Survey and Certification Group. "Centers for Medicare & Medicaid Services (CMS) Requirements for Hospital Medical Staff Privileging." Memorandum. [http://www.cms.hhs.gov/medicaid/survey-cert/sc0504.pdf]. Nov. 12, 2004.

Citizen Advocacy Center. "Improving Patient Safety and Healthcare Quality." [http://www.cacenter.org] or [http://www.4patientsafety.net]. Apr. 2002.

Citizen Advocacy Center. "What's New." [http://www.cacenter.org/new.htm]. 2004.

4PatientSafety.net. "PreP 4 Patient Safety: The Practitioner Remediation and Enhancement Partnership Pilot Project." [http://www.4patientsafety.net]. 2002.

Ginsburg, P. B., and Moy, E. "Physician Licensure and the Quality of Care: The Role of New Information Technologies." *CATO Regulation: The Review of Business and Government.* [www.cato.org/pubs/regulation]. 1992.

Institute of Medicine. *Crossing the Quality Chasm: A New Health System for the 21st Century.* Washington, D.C.: National Academies Press, 2001.

Joint Commission on Accreditation of Healthcare Organizations. *2004 Comprehensive Accreditation Manual for Hospitals.* Oakbrook Terrace, Ill.: Joint Commission on Accreditation of Healthcare Organizations, 2004a.

Joint Commission on Accreditation of Healthcare Organizations. "2004 National Patient Safety Goals." [http://www.jcaho.org/accredited+organizations/patient+safety/npsg.htm]. 2004b.

Kadzielski, M. A. "Physician and Allied Health Credentialing." In R. Carroll (ed.), *Risk Management Handbook for Health Care Organizations.* (4th ed.) Chicago: American Society for Healthcare Risk Management, 2002.

Kadzielski, M. A., and Martin, C. "Assessing Medical Error in Health Care: Controversy, Challenge, and a Culture of Safety." *Health Progress,* Nov.–Dec. 2001, *82,* 14–17.

Kadzielski, M. A., and Martin, C. "Assessing Medical Error in Health Care: Developing a 'Culture of Safety.'" *Health Progress,* Nov.–Dec. 2002, *83,* 31–35.

Kohn, L. T., Corrigan, J. M., and Donaldson, M. S. (eds.). *To Err Is Human: Building a Safer Health System.* Washington, D.C.: National Academies Press, 2000.

Larry, D., Wolfe, S. M., and Lurie, P. "Survey of Doctor Disciplinary Information on State Web Sites." Health Research Group Publication No. 1615. [http://www.citizen.org/publications]. Feb. 2000.

Leapfrog Group. "ICU Physician Staffing Factsheet." [http://www.Leapfroggroup.org]. 2003.

Leapfrog Group. "Patient Safety." [http://www.leapfroggroup.org/safety1.htm]. 2004.

National Association Medical Staff Services. *Credentialing 101: Study and Reference Guide.* Austin, Tex.: National Association Medical Staff Services, Sept. 2003.

Stewart, J. B. *Blind Eye.* New York: Simon & Schuster, 1999.

Tufts Health Plan. "Physician Group Quality Profile, Frequently Asked Questions." [http://www.tuftshealthplan.com/members/members.php?sec=quality&content=faq&rightnav=results]. 2004.

CHAPTER THIRTEEN

PLANNING FOR THE FUTURE

Fay A. Rozovsky
James R. Woods Jr.

Advances in patient safety have helped health care organizations and providers to define risk and to seek solutions. But, as with so many issues in medicine, how does one keep such an important concept from becoming a mere buzzword? From the physician who determines medical management to the pharmacist who controls distributions of prescribed medications to the nurse at the bedside, the receptionist in triage, the housekeeper, and the ward secretary, a collective effort must be made to keep the term *patient safety* from becoming just another slogan.

The naysayer might suggest that the current focus on patient safety is but the most recent iteration of quality assurance or quality improvement. The authors and editors of this book think not.

The concept of patient safety is driving a fundamental movement that will redefine the practice of medicine as a team effort and thus distinguish it from the practice of medicine in which the physician is the captain of the ship and the other care providers and assistants are there merely to carry out orders. Following this redesign, care providers will work in true collaborative relationships premised on trust, respect, and effective communication. The redesign will also encompass a change in care provider–patient relationships, so that rather than being merely recipients of care, patients will be true partners in their treatment. Likewise, recognizing the valuable role of family in the provision of health care, health care providers will envelop families in the reshaping of patient care.

Until this vision or goal is realized, problems will persist with the delivery of quality, safe patient care. Regulatory inquiries, actions, and litigation will persist in the wake of continued reports of poor care, safety concerns, and lack of leadership. A case example illustrates this point. Picture the following scenario in your hospital:

The Department of Pediatrics has just suffered through a long and complicated malpractice suit. In court, expert witnesses on both sides of the issue, some more credible than others, guided the jury members through this complicated case. Perhaps errors were made, perhaps not. In the end the expert witnesses most able to communicate with the jury, in this case the witnesses for the client, prevailed. As your organization is recovering from the multimillion-dollar settlement, the general counsel wishes to push patient safety to a visible level, a move you initiate with a noontime educational conference designed to garner a collective voice to promote this important concept. Perhaps you have brought in one or more outside speakers representing risk management and medicine. You provide food in anticipation of a large turnout. You have sent flyers out to each of the departments, extolling the importance of this educational conference.

The conference unfortunately draws only a small number of hospital employees and a few members of the medical staff. Absent are the CEO, the medical director, the chairs of the clinical departments, and the senior nurse leadership. Following the conference, you mentally disassemble the preparation and query how you can promote such an important mission in the absence of senior leadership. As you do so, all around you are the telltale signs of the underlying causes of the case that led to the multimillion-dollar settlement.

This fictional scenario is steeped in reality. Similar scenarios have played out in other health care entities such as physician groups, skilled nursing facilities, ambulatory care centers, and urgent care centers. When senior leadership does not embrace patient safety and see it as a primary driving force, little progress is made. And what does *involvement* by senior leadership mean really? Is it just authorizing the expenditure of funds? Is it hiring more staff? Is it being more aggressive in terms of weeding out "bad actors" on the nursing and medical staffs? Or does it mean rolling up one's sleeves and taking a definite stand to shift the mind-set, the culture of the health care organization?

Lessons from the Field

Several steps have been taken by medical institutions to give senior leadership a primary role in advancing the concept of patient safety. Most institutions have some form of peer review as a quality assurance activity. The dilemma for peer review and quality assurance meetings is that review usually *follows* a bad event.

This approach negates the opportunity to identify *good catches,* or *near misses,* and to examine program structures inclined to produce adverse patient events. Inroads have been made into the task of bringing the health care field into compliance with standards of acceptable practice. More can and should be done. In the meantime it is worthwhile to review what is working.

Encouraging Good Catches

The astute health care provider is apt to encounter situations in which he or she sees a potential system failure and stops it before harm occurs to a patient. Illustrations abound:

> The pharmacist who notices that the dose for a prescribed drug is too high for a pediatric patient
>
> The dietician who detects that a food-line preparer set up a full-menu tray for a "liquids only" preop patient
>
> The registered nurse who finds that "falls prevention assessment" information is lacking in the record of a long-term care facility resident with a history of orthostatic instability secondary to taking hypertensive medication
>
> The nurse anesthetist who finds a serious problem with the gas lines in the day surgery unit

In each of these examples the care provider "caught" the potential for patient injury prior to the delivery of care or service. It was a good catch. It was an early warning of a systemic failure in which various processes and subprocesses did not work properly. Like the color of the sky in the sailor's adage "Red skies in the morning, sailors take warning," the good catch informs the care provider and the health care organization that steps should be taken *now* for future safety; in health care that often means correcting systemic issues.

The good catch is different from the near miss. In the latter, harm is more narrowly averted. Most often care is just about to be provided to a patient when the error about to happen is identified and stopped. For example, elective surgery is about to begin when the operating room supervisor reports to the surgeon that a delayed set of laboratory values "rule out" the patient for surgery on the unit. That the laboratory test findings were delayed and that preparation for the operation was allowed to proceed without this set of results reflects serious systemic failures. However, that the operating room supervisor intervened with the new results turned a potential for error into a near miss. Common to near misses is the potential for a medication error. Perhaps a postoperative patient has an order for pain management written by a medical resident. The medication ordered is one to which the patient is allergic. The patient's record has a warning label on it identifying the drug allergy. Somehow the medication order process that should have alerted staff to the allergy failed, and pharmacy personnel did not detect the error. An agency nurse working on the floor is about to administer the medication when the charge nurse says, "Wait a second. Did you complete all the checks for using that medication?" Embarrassed, the agency nurse says, "Well, no, I didn't. I will do them." A couple of minutes later the agency nurse reports her findings to the charge nurse. Obviously upset, the agency nurse says, "It's a good thing you called me on that one. When I went back through the required steps, I found out that the patient was allergic to that drug."

The procedures that lead to good catches and near misses are similar to speed bumps in that each step slows down a care process, giving the health care provider time to take actions that avert error. For a good-catch or near-miss system to be effective, senior leadership must encourage it. No recrimination should be allowed against those who in good faith stop a process or report their observations.

Patient Safety Rounds

Numerous institutions have found patient safety rounds an effective vehicle for identifying near misses and discussing adverse events. For example, at the University of Rochester, borrowing from a model initiated at Johns Hopkins University, patient safety rounds are conducted monthly on each floor. In attendance are frequently the medical director, the quality assurance director, the director of pharmacy, the director of nursing, the chair of the department, and the senior nursing manager. Assembled around a table are both senior and younger care providers representing pharmacy, nursing, medicine, and operating room technical support (attendance among this group rotates monthly). In this setting individuals are encouraged to describe recent events in their own environments that potentially or actually created patient risk. These events might involve medications similarly labeled and therefore easily interchanged, care providers being summoned by beeper or phone but not responding, conflicts in conversations between a physician and a nurse in which a chain of command (a procedure for quickly resolving issues by bringing in other parties) was not apparent and therefore not used, or a diet delivered to a patient that failed to reflect the nutritional restrictions made necessary by the patient's diabetes. Each participant is told that in this forum there will be *no repercussions* for being honest, that input from each individual is valued, and that a running log of the issues raised is maintained and reviewed periodically with an eye to the resolution of issues and not just the accumulation of defects.

In the last fifteen minutes of each patient safety rounds session, the group walks onto a ward and draws ward personnel from nursing, housekeeping, and medical care to raise the same issues that the group has been discussing. Made comfortable by the promise of immunity, ward personnel can become involved in the process of discussing potential errors and seeking solutions. By rotating this type of meeting monthly on different floors in a department, senior leadership quickly recognizes areas for improvement and, most important, potential areas of adverse outcome before they can manifest themselves as real events.

Time Out

Another key practice is taking a *time out*. Rather than assuming that all is well, the collaborative team stops the care process and makes certain that all systems are in place and operational. This means that each member of the health care team must check that set of subsystems or processes for which he or she is accountable. The time-out process is particularly useful in complex situations, such as those that occur in the operating room. However, it may be just as important in other areas of the health care system. For example, it may be useful in disaster management and patient safety.

Patient Safety Is a Team Effort

Fundamental in the effort to improve patient safety has been the recognition that each individual offering care to the patient is a professional deserving of equal respect. Unlike the medical model of the early and mid-1900s, in which the physician was the boss and all other care providers were the followers, today's model features a medical team transformed into a balanced group in which each individual contributes a unique component of the total medical care the patient will receive. But how is this achieved?

First, each medical team member should be aware of the name of each of the other members. In the operating room a simple whiteboard on which all the names are written fosters familiarity within the group. Achieving such familiarity on the ward may be more challenging, as nurses attend at the patient bedside and physicians come and go, balancing their outpatient responsibilities with inpatient care. Nonetheless, acknowledging the importance of knowing each team member is a fundamental component of true patient safety.

Team building is also essential to achieving success. This may require leaders to exert considerable influence to make certain that everyone understands the importance of being a team player. Respect for other members of one's team is very important, as is the way communications are carried out among the team members. Team members must have the prerogative of disagreeing, and they should know how to disagree productively among themselves. Having a chain of command is important if team processes are to work successfully.

For many health care organizations, the collaborative team approach will mark a cultural change in the way the organization does its work. If individuals cannot work successfully in this environment, it will likely mean they have reached a point of transition in their jobs.

We All Are Human

Improving patient safety requires organizations to undergo a cultural change. The old concept was that "I am a care provider and I do not make mistakes," but the more practical philosophy is that each of us is vulnerable to making mistakes, but by working in teams and monitoring each other, we are likely to reduce our personal errors. In the team format the burden of excessive workloads and the risks of downtime place a new responsibility on good communication between team members. Absent this "glue" between team members, the culture is likely to backslide toward endorsing a more traditional and imperfect form of individual care, thus negating the value of the team. In its most developed form the team becomes a collective group of individuals, each of whom feels involved, responsible, and valued for his or her input toward improving the overall product that the team delivers. It is this effort to draw on the highest level of skill from each team member that collectively produces the most effective team.

Other Practices

A host of successful practices forge the path to change and improved patient safety. From using practice guidelines to placing greater reliance on computerized systems to making changes in staffing, methods are being designed to lessen the risk of harm to patients and to enhance compliance with regulatory and accreditation requirements.

Creating a zone in which health care as a field can incubate innovations is important. Rather than inhabiting an atmosphere that is punitive, prescriptive, and driven by regulatory compliance, health care organizations and providers need the opportunity to invent new systems and to enhance existing structures to achieve safety. Input from the end user, including the patient, is essential in this regard. Once again, leadership must take action to transform the system to enable such innovation.

Conclusion: The Future Depends on Leadership

If patient safety is going to become an enduring and primary goal, it will take more than money, personnel, and legislative change. It will require leaders willing to bite the bullet and to change the way health care services are provided along the continuum of care. Leadership must act in a decisive, accountable, responsible manner. Legislation and regulation set minimum norms or expectations. To go beyond that, much has to come from within the health care field and from individual service providers. Many fine suggestions for achieving patient safety and quality care have been posited in this book. What will it take to make patient safety a reality? Here are some ideas for the future:

Design leadership education. Boards, policy analysts, legislators, and regulators need specific education on their roles and responsibilities in patient safety.

Work to inform patients and family members. Rather than assuming patients and their loved ones know what is expected of them, health care organizations and providers must inform them in a way that is meaningful, understandable, and respectful. Moreover, patients and their families need a demonstrable voice in patient safety.

Provide tools and training. Health care providers and institutions need practical tools and materials to get their jobs done correctly. Equipment with fail-safes is essential, as are demonstrated competencies in using the equipment.

Learn from error. Rather than treating adverse events or systems failures as isolated events, we need to collect outcomes, analyze them, and use the findings to redesign systems and to educate care providers and patients alike. Making this commonplace will require a hefty change in legislative attitudes toward evidentiary protection and in the use of such findings as a sword during malpractice litigation or professional disciplinary action.

Embrace accountability. The health care system and health care providers must embrace accountability. No system is blame-free and no care provider is a wholly innocent party. Finger pointing is of little utility. Helping the care provider who lacks competencies is important. However, removing the care provider who is a risk to patients and others from the delivery system is a responsibility of leadership in an accountable organization.

Health care is poised for dramatic change. Such change is needed now if patient safety is to become a reality.

INDEX